Motivational Interviewing for Hospice and Palliative Care

Communication Skills for End-of-Life Conversations, Goals of Care, and Family Support

Clarissa Mary Fernandez

Motivational Interviewing for Hospice an

This book is intended for general informational and educational purposes. It is not a substitute for professional training, clinical judgment, individualized supervision, or direct medical, legal, psychological, or ethical guidance. Readers should rely on their own professional expertise and the policies of their employing institutions when applying any concept or practice discussed in these pages.

No outcomes are guaranteed. Clinical communication is shaped by factors that no single text can capture, and no technique described here will produce specific results in every situation. Readers are responsible for their own clinical decisions, their own practice, and the consequences of applying what they read.

All patients, families, and clinicians portrayed in the scenarios and examples within this book are composite or fictionalized. Any resemblance to real persons, living or deceased, is coincidental. Names, roles, and circumstances have been used illustratively and are not intended to harm, misrepresent, or identify any real individual, family, or institution.

First Edition, 2026.

ISBN: 978-1-7646390-2-6

Table of Contents

Preface

Most books about end-of-life communication prescribe what to say. This one attends to how to listen.

The field of hospice and palliative care has been shaped, over the past five decades, by remarkable advances in symptom management, ethics, and interdisciplinary practice. What has lagged behind is the discipline of the conversation itself. Clinicians graduate from nursing, medical, social work, and divinity schools with solid grounding in the clinical dimensions of end of life care, and almost no training in the communicative skill that serves as the vehicle for all of it. The result is a generation of capable practitioners who walk into the hardest rooms of their careers without a shared framework for the talking.

The usual response to this gap has been communication training. Workshops on breaking bad news. Modules on cultural competency. Webinars on goals of care conversations. These efforts are useful and insufficient. They teach phrases to say without attending to the underlying craft of engagement. They instruct clinicians in what good communication looks like without giving them a way to produce it under the pressure of the bedside. A clinician who has attended three such trainings is often left with the same uncomfortable gap between the seminar room and the kitchen table at midnight where a widow cannot bring herself to give her husband the morphine.

Motivational interviewing, developed by William Miller and Stephen Rollnick across three decades of clinical research and practice, offers something different. It is not a list of phrases. It is a disciplined method for engaging people who are ambivalent, frightened, or in the middle of decisions they do not feel equipped to make. The evidence base for MI in addiction treatment, health behavior change, chronic disease management, and mental health is substantial. Its adaptation for hospice and palliative care, while emerging in the clinical literature since the early 2000s, has not until now been given the depth of treatment that working clinicians need.

The present volume is that treatment. It takes the full architecture of motivational interviewing, including the spirit of MI, the four processes of engaging, focusing, evoking, and planning, the OARS skills of open questions, affirmations, reflections, and summaries, and the fidelity benchmarks that distinguish proficient practice, and applies them chapter by chapter to the specific conversations that define end of life work. The conversation about hospice that the patient keeps refusing. The prognosis question the clinician does not want to answer. The family meeting that is about to fragment. The caregiver who freezes at the medication. The absent relative who arrives demanding a reversal. The child asking if they are going to die.

The approach is practical rather than theoretical. Each chapter opens with a clinical scene, develops the relevant MI skills against that scene, works through specific scripts and moves, demonstrates the skills in extended worked examples, and closes with the failure modes that experienced clinicians will recognize. The writing assumes the reader is working. The scenarios are drawn from the actual textures of hospice, palliative, and end of life practice. The research is cited precisely and without flourish.

The book is structured in six parts. Part One establishes the foundations: the problem the book addresses, the spirit of MI, the nature of ambivalence, and the question of when to guide versus when to follow. Part Two develops the core OARS skills for end of life settings. Part Three walks through the toughest conversations: introducing hospice, breaking bad news, discussing prognosis, developing goals of care that hold, working with feared medications, and navigating decisions about food, water, and treatment. Part Four addresses family dynamics: meetings, disagreements, and the late arriving relative. Part Five considers special populations: dementia care, pediatric palliative practice, and cultural context. Part Six closes with the sustainability of the clinician doing this work, including attention to cumulative grief and team culture. Seven appendices provide a pocket card, annotated scenarios, a walk through of the Serious Illness Conversation Guide, a self assessment tool, team exercises, family handouts, and curated references for continued learning.

What this book aims to give the reader is not a set of phrases to memorize. It is a coherent framework for the conversational work of end of life care, grounded in evidence, illustrated in practice, and usable in the rooms where the reader will find themselves next week. The chapters that follow are organized around the real questions that clinicians bring to this work: how to open, how to hear, how to hold difficult content, how to move toward decisions without forcing them, how to stay present across time, and how to sustain oneself while doing any of it. The craft is learnable. The evidence supports its effect on patient outcomes, family bereavement, and clinician wellbeing. What remains is the work of developing the skill in the specific hands of the specific clinician reading these pages.

That work begins in the next chapter.

PART I: FOUNDATIONS

Chapter 1: Why Good Clinicians Struggle Here

Dr. Miguel Ortega had been practicing oncology for nineteen years. He had sat on tumor boards for every subtype of breast cancer you could name. He walked patients through third line therapy options with the steadiness of a clinician who knew the data cold. When colleagues needed a second opinion on a complex case, they called Miguel.

On a Tuesday in March, Miguel stood in an exam room with Mrs. Tanaka and her daughter Amara. Mrs. Tanaka's metastatic pancreatic cancer had progressed through two lines of chemotherapy. The scans from last week showed new liver lesions. Miguel had the conversation laid out in his head. He would explain that further treatment was unlikely to extend her life and that hospice could provide excellent symptom management and support. He had given some version of this talk hundreds of times.

He opened his mouth and heard himself say, "Given the radiographic progression and your declining performance status, I think we should consider transitioning toward a more conservative approach with emphasis on symptom directed interventions and perhaps involvement of the supportive care team."

Mrs. Tanaka nodded slowly. Amara stared at him.

"Does that mean she's going to die?" Amara asked.

Miguel felt the heat rise in his chest. He tried again. "Well, the trajectory of the disease suggests that further aggressive measures may not be in her best interest, and we want to prioritize quality of life at this point."

He could hear himself, and he hated what he heard. He was a clinician who had held his own son's hand at his best friend's funeral. He was not a man who hid from hard truths. Yet here, in this room, with this woman who had trusted him for two years, he had hidden behind the same jargon he mocked when residents used it.

This chapter is about why the conversation you just witnessed happens so often. Not to you specifically, but across the field. You will see the training gap that nobody mentions in medical school or nursing orientation. You will learn why the most popular bad news protocols only get you halfway there. You will find out who actually does most of the talking in palliative consultations, and why that matters. By the end, you will have language for your own struggle and a clear sense of what needs to change.

1.1 The Training Gap

Miguel graduated from medical school with over 200 hours of training in pharmacology, close to that in pathology, and somewhere around six total hours dedicated to end of life communication. Those six hours covered breaking bad news, advance care planning, and cultural considerations. Combined. That is the norm, not the outlier.

The numbers vary by institution and specialty, but the pattern is consistent. A national survey of oncologists found that 57 percent felt inadequately trained in prognostication (Lamont and Christakis, 2001). A more recent inpatient oncology study also identified substantial barriers to goals-of-care conversations among clinicians caring for hospitalized patients with cancer (Wheless et al., 2023). Most internal medicine residents report feeling unprepared to discuss hospice referral by the time they finish residency (Sullivan et al., 2003). Communication scholarship in palliative nursing describes similar deficits in end-of-life communication training and preparedness (Wittenberg-Lyles et al., 2008).

You did not fail your training. Your training failed you.

Here is what the gap looks like in practice. You learned the Krebs cycle by diagramming it seventeen times. You memorized the brachial plexus by quizzing yourself until you could recite it on command. When you were ready to try a central line, someone stood behind you and coached your hands. You practiced listening to heart sounds on standardized patients and got feedback on what you heard. You practiced suturing on pig feet.

Then, on the third floor of a teaching hospital, someone handed you a chart and said, "Go tell Mr. Delmonico's family that the cancer has spread."

There was no standardized patient for that. No corrected repetitions. No attending watching you pace the words and asking you to try again with a softer opening. You did your best. You went back to your charting. Nobody reviewed what you said. If you did it badly, you probably never found out. If you did it well, that also went unmarked.

Communication is a clinical skill. It responds to deliberate practice the way everything else does. Clinicians who receive structured communication training show measurable improvements in rapport, information giving, and response to patient emotion (Moore et al., 2018; Back et al., 2007). The reason most of your colleagues still struggle is not a deficit of empathy or intelligence. It is a deficit of practice with feedback. That is fixable.

1.2 Why Protocols Stop Short

Most clinicians who have had any end of life communication training have met **SPIKES**, the six step protocol for breaking bad news developed by Robert Buckman and colleagues (Baile et al., 2000). Setting. Perception. Invitation. Knowledge. Emotions. Strategy. It is a sturdy framework and it has helped thousands of trainees get past the panic of the first conversation.

But SPIKES does not teach you what to do when the patient says "I feel so good today, maybe I shouldn't enroll in hospice."

SPIKES does not teach you what to do when the daughter says she wants everything done while the son says his father never wanted to live like this.

SPIKES does not teach you how to sit with a widow who wants to keep spoon feeding her dying husband even though he is aspirating.

SPIKES is a bad news delivery protocol. It gets you into the conversation. It does not get you through the conversation. For the hundred other moments that make up hospice and palliative care practice, you need a different set of tools.

This is the gap that **Motivational Interviewing** fills. MI is not a protocol. It is a way of being with another person that produces a set of specific skills. Those skills apply to every conversation where the patient or family is ambivalent, resistant, overwhelmed, or grieving. Which, in palliative care, is every conversation.

The original MI researchers, William Miller and Stephen Rollnick, built the approach for substance use counseling in the 1980s. Over the past two decades, clinicians have adapted it for primary care, diabetes management, medication adherence, and, more recently, palliative care (Pollak et al., 2011). The adaptation is not automatic. Some of the classical MI machinery, like decisional balance or planning scales, was built for behavior change and does not fit end of life work neatly. But the spirit of MI, and the core skills of open questions, affirmations, reflections, and summaries, translate beautifully into this setting.

You do not need to throw out SPIKES. You need to build what comes after it.

1.3 A Real Example

Meet Elena. She was a palliative care nurse practitioner in her fourth year, working in a community hospital in Albuquerque. She had done SPIKES training in fellowship. She could set the scene, ask permission, deliver the news, and manage the immediate emotional response with real grace.

Last spring, she was called to consult on a 72 year old man with end stage heart failure. His cardiologist had recommended hospice. The patient refused. The cardiologist asked Elena to "try to talk him into it."

Elena walked in with SPIKES running in her head. She set up. She asked what he understood. She laid out the medical picture. She acknowledged his emotions. At the end, she asked if he would reconsider hospice.

He said no.

She left the room frustrated. She had done the protocol, and the protocol had given her nothing for the moment after he said no.

That night she pulled up an article on MI in palliative care and read it twice. The next morning she went back. This time she did not try to convince him of anything. She asked, "Tell me what a good day looks like for you now."

He talked for twenty minutes. He told her about his granddaughter's wedding coming up in April. He told her about how he hated the ER and never wanted to go back. He told her he did not know what hospice actually was.

By the end of the conversation, he had asked her to explain what hospice would look like at home. He did not sign up that day. He did three days later.

What this means for you: The reason your first conversation did not work is not always that you used the wrong words. Sometimes it is that you tried to deliver the information before you understood what the patient was actually worried about. MI gives you a way to find that out before you deliver anything.

1.4 Who Is Actually Talking

Here is a pattern researchers keep finding when they record palliative care conversations. Across multiple studies of oncology and palliative care visits, clinicians speak somewhere between 60 and 75 percent of the time (Tulsky et al., 2011; Singh et al., 2017). The patient and family talk the rest.

Read that again. The people facing death, and the people who love them, get one third of the airtime in the conversation that is supposed to be about their lives.

This is not because clinicians are bad listeners. It is because clinicians are trained to deliver information. We explain disease. We explain prognosis. We explain options. When we run out of information to deliver, we feel awkward, so we deliver more. Silence feels like failure. So we fill it.

The problem is that people process bad news in their own time. When you fill the silence, you rob them of the moment they needed to absorb what you just said. Worse, you never find out what they were actually thinking. You walk out of the room confident you have "explained it well" and the family walks out of the room with a tenth of what they needed to know.

One study of oncology consultations found that when a patient expressed an emotional cue (a sigh, a worried question, a trailing off), clinicians responded to the emotion with empathy only 22 percent of the time. Most of the time they redirected to medical content (Morse et al., 2008). The patient's emotion got parked. The clinician felt productive. Neither of them got what they needed.

The 70 percent problem is not solved by talking less. It is solved by asking differently. Open questions that surface what the patient is thinking. Reflections that show you heard what they said. Silences that are offered as gifts rather than gaps to fill. These are MI skills, and they can flip the ratio without making you feel like you abandoned your clinical role.

1.5 What Families Remember

Five years from now, the Tanaka family will not remember Miguel's words about "radiographic progression" or "conservative approach." They will not remember the exam room or the weather that day or the time on the clock. What they will remember is if Miguel seemed to see their mother as a person or as a case.

Bereaved family members interviewed years after a loved one's death tend to report remarkably consistent things about their clinicians. They remember moments of presence. They remember being listened to without being rushed. They remember a nurse who sat down. They remember a physician who cried. They remember the person who said their mother's name correctly on every visit (Virdun et al., 2015; Heyland et al., 2010).

They also remember the harms. They remember the doctor who would not make eye contact. They remember the nurse who answered every question with a brochure. They remember the resident who used the word "expired." These memories do not fade with time. For many bereaved families, the quality of end of life communication predicts their mental health outcomes for years afterward (Wright et al., 2008).

This is not an argument for being extra warm at the end of life. It is an argument for understanding what this conversation actually is. You are not delivering data. You are participating in a moment that the family will carry for the rest of their lives. That changes the calculation. It changes what skill looks like.

MI is not a softer way to talk. It is a more accurate way to talk, for a situation where accuracy about words and procedures matters less than accuracy about people.

1.6 Another Real Example

Meet Raj. He was a hospice medical director in his eighth year when he took over a struggling home hospice program in rural Georgia. His admission rate was fine. His length of stay was terrible. Patients were dying within days of enrollment because their families were referring them too late.

He figured the fix was education. He made a slide deck about hospice eligibility. He drove it around to five local primary care clinics. He watched a lot of doctors nod politely.

Nothing changed.

In month six he tried something different. Instead of teaching, he started asking. He invited the referring physicians to fifteen minute conversations. He asked what made them hesitate to mention hospice earlier. He asked what they worried about when they did.

What he heard surprised him. The doctors were not confused about eligibility. They were scared of the conversation itself. They were afraid patients would think they were "giving up" on them. They were afraid families would be angry. They had tried it a few times and it had gone badly and they had stopped trying.

Raj did not argue. He listened. He reflected back what he heard. Then he asked one more question: "If I could come with you to one of those conversations, would you be interested?"

Eleven of the fifteen doctors said yes. Over the next year, his median length of stay doubled. Not because he taught differently. Because he asked differently.

What this means for you: MI works on the people you work with, not only on patients and families. The same skills that open a conversation with a scared patient open a conversation with a scared colleague. When you stop trying to convince and start trying to understand, change follows.

1.7 A New Posture

The word "posture" matters. Communication skill at end of life is not primarily about what comes out of your mouth. It is about how you are standing, emotionally, before you say anything at all.

Clinicians trained in traditional bad news models tend to adopt a posture that researchers call the **expert stance**. You have the information. You deliver it. You manage the emotional response. You move on to the plan. It is a posture that has served medicine well in acute care and procedural work. It fails in palliative care because the situation is not primarily informational.

The MI posture is different. It is collaborative rather than expert. It assumes the patient and family know things you do not know, specifically about what matters to them and what they can handle. It assumes your job is to understand those things before you offer anything, and sometimes in place of offering anything. It treats silence as useful, emotion as data, and ambivalence as normal.

This does not mean you abandon your medical knowledge or your clinical judgment. Miguel still knew more about pancreatic cancer than Mrs. Tanaka's family did. Elena still knew more about hospice than her patient did. The difference is what you do with that knowledge. In the expert stance, you deliver it. In the MI stance, you make it available when it serves the patient's own thinking.

This book is about building that posture and the skills that flow from it. It is not a replacement for SPIKES or for the Serious Illness Conversation Guide or for any of the other frameworks you already use. It is the undercarriage that makes those frameworks work in real conversations with real people who are facing the hardest moment of their lives.

The rest of this book is practical. You will meet specific skills, specific scripts, specific situations. You will see what MI looks like in a nursing home on a Tuesday afternoon and in an ICU at 2 a.m.

You will see how to use these skills in a fifteen minute home visit and in a ninety minute family meeting. The theory stops here. Starting in Chapter 2.0, you will be inside the work.

1.8 When It Does Not Work

The most common way clinicians fail at this early on is that they try to hold an MI posture and deliver complex medical content in the same breath. They ask a beautiful open question, get a rich answer, and then immediately start lecturing about opioid pharmacology or hospice eligibility or whatever their original agenda was. The patient feels the shift from "you are listening" to "you are selling" and shuts down.

This is not a character flaw. It is a reflex. You have a limited visit, you have information you believe the family needs, and the minute you stop actively listening, your clinician brain reaches for the data. Over and over, new MI learners describe the same feeling: "I was doing well and then I blew it by giving the speech."

Three things to try when this happens to you:

1. Write down the three or four pieces of information you feel you must communicate before you walk into the room. If there are more than four, cross off the bottom half. Now you have space to ask. 2. When you hear yourself start to explain, pause. Ask a question instead. The explanation will still be there in two minutes. 3. End the visit with the question "What else do you want to ask me about today?" rather than a summary of what you told them. This gives you one more look at what they actually heard.

If you find you are still explaining more than asking after a month of trying, it might help to have a colleague observe one of your conversations and tell you where you slipped. That is harder than reading a book about it. It is also the single fastest way to change.

1.9 The Quick Version

Most clinicians who struggle with end of life conversations were trained exhaustively in everything except those conversations. You are not bad at this because you are a bad clinician. You are rusty because nobody gave you deliberate practice with feedback. SPIKES and similar protocols get you in the door. They do not carry you through the twenty other moments where the conversation actually happens.

Research shows clinicians do about 70 percent of the talking in palliative consultations, miss most emotional cues, and underestimate how much families remember about the tone of these conversations years later. Families remember your presence or your absence far more than they remember your words.

The alternative is a different posture. Not expert delivering news, but companion surfacing what matters. That posture has a name and a set of skills. It is called Motivational Interviewing, adapted for this setting. You will meet it properly in the next chapter, starting with what its founders call "the spirit of MI," which is the part that has to come before the skills or the skills do nothing.

Chapter 2: The Spirit Beneath The Skills

Ellen was a social work intern on her second week at a home hospice program in New Orleans. Her supervisor had partnered her with a nurse for a home visit to see Betty, an eighty year old woman whose husband Frank was dying of prostate cancer. The visit was supposed to be straightforward. Orient Betty to the hospice plan. Assess for caregiver burden. Drop off a packet of pamphlets.

When Betty opened the door the next morning, Ellen almost did not recognize her. The day before, Betty had been neatly dressed and composed. Today her clothes were rumpled, her hair flat on one side, bags under her eyes like bruises. The nurse had called ahead to ask Ellen to come alone. Betty had been trying to spoon feed Frank even though he could barely swallow. The nurse had explained the risks. Betty had not wanted to hear it. The nurse thought Betty was being difficult.

Ellen sat on the couch. She had one tool from her graduate course in motivational interviewing, and she had not used it in the field yet. She asked Betty how the night had been. Betty told her. She talked about Frank moaning at 3 a.m. and how scared she had been. Ellen did not correct anything. She did not teach anything. She reflected what she heard: "It sounds like you have been loving him with everything you have, and you are exhausted."

Betty started to cry. Then she started to talk, really talk, about the sixty four years of meals she had made for this man. About the Sunday roast that had been their first meal as a married couple. About what food meant between them. By the end of the visit, Betty was the one who said the feeding might not be the way to love him anymore. She was not ready to stop. But she was ready to talk about it.

Ellen walked to her car and sat in the driver's seat for ten minutes. She had not explained anything. She had not taught anything. She had used a single reflection. And something had opened that had been closed the day before.

This chapter is about what Ellen did, and what she did not do, and why the difference matters. You will meet the four principles that make up the **spirit of MI**, the part that has to be present before any of the techniques can work. You will see why clinicians who learn the skills without the spirit often make things worse. You will also see what the spirit looks like in a hospice setting, which is different from what it looks like in substance use counseling where MI was born.

2.1 Partnership Over Expertise

Miller and Rollnick, who developed MI, describe its spirit in four words: partnership, acceptance, compassion, and evocation (Miller and Rollnick, 2023). The first of these, partnership, is the posture you stand in before the conversation even starts.

Partnership means you do not walk into the room as the person with the answers. You walk in as someone who has clinical expertise and is about to meet an expert on a different subject: the patient or family in front of you, who are the only people who know what their lives, values, and capacities actually are.

This is not false modesty. You do know more about disease trajectories, about what hospice covers, about what opioid titration looks like, about what happens in the last 48 hours. That knowledge matters. The question is what you do with it. In the expert stance, you lead with it. In the partnership stance, you hold it in reserve and bring it forward when it serves the patient's own thinking.

Ellen did not walk into Betty's living room thinking she had the answer. She did not know what the right answer was. She suspected continuing to feed Frank was medically risky. She also suspected it was the last way Betty knew how to tell him she loved him. Those two things sat next to each other. Ellen's job was not to pick one. It was to help Betty see both clearly and let Betty do her own picking.

Partnership shows up in small behaviors. You sit down rather than stand. You ask permission before you explain something. You say "what do you think" before you say "what I think." You tolerate answers you did not expect. You do not interrupt. When you do not know what to say, you do not say anything, instead of filling the air with something clinical.

These behaviors sound simple. In an exam room, under time pressure, with three more patients waiting, they are not simple at all. Partnership is a discipline. It has to be chosen again every visit.

2.2 Acceptance As A Stance

The second element of MI spirit is **acceptance**, which Miller and Rollnick break into four components: absolute worth, accurate empathy, autonomy support, and affirmation. In end of life work, these four matter in specific ways.

Absolute worth means you treat every patient and family member as having value that does not depend on their decisions. The patient who refuses hospice has the same worth as the patient who signs up. The son who wants aggressive treatment for his dying mother has the same worth as the one who wants comfort care. You do not reward agreement with warmth and punish disagreement with distance. This is easier said than done when you are tired and they are the fourth difficult family this week.

Accurate empathy means your job is to understand what the person is experiencing from the inside, not to make them feel better from the outside. This is a distinction that escapes many kind clinicians. Making someone feel better is about you, about relieving the discomfort you feel when they are suffering. Understanding them accurately is about them. It sometimes increases their distress in the short term because it means naming what they are actually feeling rather than reaching for a reassurance that moves past it.

Autonomy support means you protect their right to make their own decisions even when you disagree. This is not passive. It is active respect. It means asking "Would you like my thoughts on that?" before you give them. It means saying "This is your call" and meaning it.

Affirmation is not flattery. It is specific, grounded recognition of strengths and effort you have actually observed. "You are doing a great job" is empty. "You learned how to reposition him by yourself in one afternoon" is affirmation. The first reassures the clinician that they are being supportive. The second tells the caregiver something true about themselves.

2.3 Compassion That Is Not Rescue

The third element is compassion. This word has been watered down by wellness industries. In MI, compassion has a precise meaning: pursuing the welfare of the other person as an end in itself, not as a means to your own satisfaction.

The difference matters because a lot of what looks like compassion in clinical work is actually rescue, and rescue has a different flavor. Rescue is what happens when you cannot tolerate the other person's pain and you reach for a fix to stop it. The fix is often for you, not for them. A family member is crying; you hand them a tissue and say "everything is going to be okay." That is rescue. The tissue was for them. The "everything is going to be okay" was for you.

Compassion sits with the pain. It does not rush. It tolerates the fact that you cannot fix it. Paradoxically, compassion often leads to better clinical decisions than rescue does, because it does not push the conversation forward before the patient is ready.

Consider two responses to a daughter who says "I can't believe this is happening to her." The rescue response: "I know this is hard, but your mother is comfortable and we are taking very good care of her." The compassionate response: "You can't believe it. Tell me what you mean." The rescue response closes the door. The compassionate response opens it.

This is hard for clinicians trained to fix. Sitting with unresolved suffering feels like failure. It is not. It is often the single most therapeutic thing you can do. Bereavement researchers have found that families who felt their clinicians sat with them during the hardest moments report better grief outcomes years later, regardless of if anything was fixed (Kissane and Parnes, 2014).

2.4 Evocation Without Right Answers

The fourth element is **evocation**. This is the MI principle that the motivation to change, or the values that guide a hard decision, already live inside the patient. Your job is to draw them out, not to install them.

In substance use counseling, where MI was born, this meant evoking the person's own reasons to quit drinking rather than listing reasons for them. In hospice, the application is different because there is often no "change" in the behavior sense. The patient is dying. The "change" is often accepting that, or deciding how to live in it, or figuring out what they want the last weeks to look like.

Evocation in this setting means trusting that the patient and family have their own values, and that your job is to help those values come to the surface where they can guide decisions. The values may not match yours. You may think the family is making the wrong choice. Evocation asks you to bracket that and help them get to clarity on their own terms.

This is the part of MI that feels hardest to clinicians at first. You have an opinion about what is medically appropriate. You believe, correctly, that continued chemotherapy in a patient with days to live is harmful. Evocation does not ask you to pretend you do not believe this. It asks you to let the patient and family arrive at their own conclusion, with your help but not with your conclusion handed to them.

There is a place for directive input in palliative care; Chapter 4.0 will walk through when to give it. For now, the principle is: lead with evocation. Most of the time, the family already has the information they need. What they are stuck on is not knowing what they think.

2.5 Spirit And Skills Together

Here is a pattern that plays out in every MI training program. A clinician learns the four skills, usually called **OARS**: open questions, affirmations, reflections, and summaries. They start using them. They ask an open question. They give an affirmation. And the conversation gets worse.

What went wrong is that they did the skills without the spirit. They asked an open question because the training told them to, not because they actually wanted to know the answer. They gave an affirmation because the training said to, not because they had actually noticed something to affirm. The patient feels the difference immediately, even if they cannot name it. What they feel is a clinician following a script. It is worse than no MI at all, because it has the surface features of attention without the reality of it.

Skills without spirit is theater. It sometimes fools the clinician but rarely fools the patient.

The opposite also matters. Spirit without skills is often just a kind person flailing. You can care deeply about a patient and still have no idea how to handle the moment when they say "I want to stop eating." Caring is necessary but not sufficient. The skills give you structure for what to do when the moment arrives. They are how the caring becomes useful instead of stuck.

The goal of this book is to build both in parallel. Each chapter from here forward introduces a specific skill or scenario, grounded in the spirit you just met. When you try a skill and it does not work, the first question to ask yourself is usually not "did I use the right words" but "was I actually in partnership with this person, or was I performing partnership while trying to get them to an outcome."

2.6 A Real Example

Meet Marcus. He was a chaplain at a large cancer center in Chicago, eleven years into his work. He was known among the staff for being quiet in family meetings. Other chaplains sometimes teased him for how little he said. The nurses knew better.

On a Thursday, Marcus was called to a family meeting for a 58 year old woman with metastatic breast cancer who was declining rapidly. Her husband Hassan and her three adult children were there. The oncologist presented the medical picture. The palliative care doctor discussed hospice. The social worker walked through logistics. Everyone looked at Marcus.

Marcus said, "I am hearing a lot of information, and I am wondering what you are all thinking."

There was a long silence. The oldest daughter spoke first. She talked about how her mother had always been the one who held the family together. The son said he was not ready. Hassan said nothing.

Marcus said to Hassan, "You have not said much."

Hassan looked at him for a long moment, then said, "I don't know who I am without her." And he cried.

Marcus did not say anything. He put his hand on Hassan's shoulder. The three children moved closer. They sat like that for maybe two minutes. When the silence broke, it was Hassan who spoke. He said, "Okay. I think we need to do this hospice thing. She would not want to be in here anymore."

Marcus had said fewer than twenty words in the entire meeting.

What this means for you: Spirit is not a feeling. It is a discipline. Marcus was not waiting for inspiration. He was actively holding space, actively refusing to fill the silence, actively trusting that the family knew what they needed to say if he gave them room to say it. That is a skill. It looks like quiet but it is not passive.

2.7 Another Real Example

Meet Isabella. She was a hospice nurse in her first year. She had taken a weekend MI workshop three weeks before. She was trying to use what she learned on every visit.

On a Tuesday morning she went to see Mr. Patel, a 79 year old man with end stage COPD. He was on continuous oxygen. His wife was caring for him at home. Isabella had a list of teaching points she wanted to cover: oxygen safety, sign of dying, when to call the hospice line.

She walked in and asked Mr. Patel an open question: "How have you been feeling this week?"

He said, "Not good."

She said, "Tell me more about that."

He said, "I am tired. I am ready."

Isabella panicked. She had been told in training that this was a cue for reflection. She said, "You are tired." Then she could not think of what to say next, so she started her teaching points about oxygen safety. Mr. Patel stared out the window. His wife looked away. The visit ended badly.

That afternoon Isabella called her preceptor and described what had happened. Her preceptor asked her a question: "What did you actually want to know when you asked him how he was feeling?"

Isabella said, "I wanted to know how his breathing was so I could adjust his medications."

Her preceptor said, "Then that is what you should have asked. Open questions are not a trick to get people to open up. They are a way to ask what you actually want to know. If you did not want to know what Mr. Patel meant by 'ready,' you should not have invited him to tell you."

Isabella went back the next week. This time she asked only what she actually wanted to know. The visit was more ordinary. It was also more honest.

What this means for you: Spirit means you ask questions whose answers you are prepared to receive. If you are not ready to hear that a patient is ready to die, do not ask a question that might surface that answer, because when he gives it, you will panic and retreat, and you will have done more harm than if you had stuck to clinical signs.

2.8 When It Does Not Work

The most common failure mode with spirit is that you forget it is a stance, not a technique. You read a chapter like this one, you feel inspired, you go into your next visit determined to be in partnership and show compassion and evoke values. Ninety seconds in, you hit a moment of pressure, and your old patterns take over. You start explaining. You give advice they did not ask for. You offer reassurance to quiet your own discomfort.

This is not a sign you failed. It is a sign you are human. The clinicians who get better at this are not the ones who never slip. They are the ones who notice the slip sooner and return to the stance.

Three things to try when you feel yourself slipping:

1. Before your next visit, take thirty seconds in the hallway to remember you are walking in to learn what the patient is experiencing, not to deliver anything. That single reset can reshape the first five minutes. 2. When you catch yourself explaining something they did not ask about, stop mid sentence. Say, "Let me come back to that. What are you thinking right now?" It is awkward and it works. 3. Debrief one conversation a week with a colleague. Not a case conference. A five minute "here is how I actually felt in that room" conversation. This is where the real learning happens.

If you notice that you cannot hold the stance for more than a minute, it is worth asking what is happening inside you. Sometimes the issue is not technique. It is that you are burned out, or you are carrying unprocessed grief from a recent death, or you are afraid of something in this particular patient. Chapter 22.0 covers that. For now, know that the stance is hard and it gets easier, and dropping it is ordinary and not a failure.

2.9 What To Take Away

The spirit of MI is the four part posture you bring into the room: partnership with the patient as expert on their own life, acceptance of their worth and autonomy, compassion that sits with suffering instead of fixing it, and evocation that trusts what is already inside them. This posture has to be present before the skills can work. Without it, the skills feel like manipulation. Without the skills, the posture has nowhere to go.

Ellen, the social work intern, changed a conversation about feeding with a single reflection because she was actually in partnership, actually compassionate, actually evoking. Marcus, the chaplain, changed a family meeting by saying almost nothing, because his silence was a form of active presence rather than absence. Isabella, the new hospice nurse, stumbled when she used the skills without the stance, and got better when she started asking questions whose answers she was prepared to receive.

The next chapter moves into the most specific feature of end of life conversations, the one that makes this work different from everything else you do. That feature is ambivalence. Patients and families facing death are almost always of two minds about what they want. Learning to work with ambivalence, rather than against it, is the heart of MI in this setting.

Chapter 3: Ambivalence Is The Point

It was 2:15 on a Wednesday afternoon when Nicole, a home hospice nurse, sat down across from Mr. Delacroix in his living room. She had been the nurse on his case for six days. He was 67, with metastatic lung cancer, on home hospice after a two week inpatient stay. His pain was controlled. His oxygen saturation was better than it had been in months. He had walked from his bedroom to the couch without the walker that morning for the first time in a week.

He said to her, "I feel so good today. Maybe I shouldn't be on hospice."

Nicole had heard some version of this sentence more times than she could count. Every hospice nurse has. On the surface it sounds like the patient is second guessing the decision. What is actually happening is something more subtle and more common.

Nicole knew the right answer was not to correct him. She also knew the right answer was not to agree with him. She said, "You are feeling strong today. And that makes hospice harder to think about."

Mr. Delacroix looked at her. He said, "Yeah. I mean, why am I giving up if this is how I feel today?"

Nicole said, "You wonder if this morning means the cancer is not as bad as we said. And at the same time, you remember the weeks before you came into the hospital."

He was quiet for a while. Then he said, "Both things are true, right? I feel better right now and I am still dying."

Nicole said, "Yes."

That is a conversation about ambivalence handled well. It did not resolve anything. Mr. Delacroix did not sign a new form. He did not commit to staying on hospice. He walked through a moment of doubt and came out the other side with a clearer picture of what he was actually living with. That is what MI in this setting usually looks like. Not dramatic conversions. Small moments of internal clarity.

This chapter is about ambivalence at end of life, which is different from ambivalence in other clinical settings. You will learn what it looks like, why it is almost always present, and why the natural clinician response of trying to "resolve" it often makes things worse. You will learn the MI language of sustain talk and change talk, adapted for a setting where the change is often acceptance rather than behavior. And you will see why pushing through ambivalence, even with the best intentions, backfires every time.

3.1 Ambivalence Near Death

Ambivalence is the experience of wanting two things at once, especially two things that cannot both be true. I want to stop the chemo because it is killing me. I also want to keep the chemo because stopping feels like giving up. Both sentences are real. Both sentences are spoken by the same patient, sometimes in the same visit, sometimes in the same breath.

In most clinical settings, ambivalence is a stage you pass through. The patient with chronic pain is ambivalent about starting opioids; with good counseling, they resolve it, and start. The patient with depression is ambivalent about medication; with education, they resolve it, and take it. The clinician's job is to help resolve the ambivalence in a direction that serves the patient.

In end of life care, the ambivalence rarely resolves. Not because the patient is stuck but because both sides of the ambivalence are permanently true.

Mr. Delacroix is dying and today he feels good. Those are not contradictions to be resolved. They are simultaneous facts. The patient who enrolls in hospice is both relieved and devastated. The family member who makes the decision to withdraw ventilation is both at peace and destroyed. Trying to talk them into feeling only one of these things is not just ineffective, it is dismissive of what is actually happening to them.

This is why standard decisional tools, like pros and cons lists, often feel wrong here. A pros and cons list assumes there is a decision to be made that will then settle the matter. Near death, the decision has usually already been made by the disease. What the patient is wrestling with is how to hold what they cannot change.

Ambivalence at end of life is not a problem. It is the normal state. The clinician's job is not to fix it. The clinician's job is to help the patient carry it.

3.2 Existential Versus Behavioral

Classical MI grew up treating **behavioral ambivalence**. Do I keep drinking or quit? Do I take the medication or not? Do I go to the AA meeting or stay home? The behavior is the unit. The change is observable. The ambivalence has a resolution, even if reaching it takes time.

Existential ambivalence is different. It is not about a behavior. It is about how to stand in relation to a reality you cannot change. Do I accept that I am dying, or keep fighting? Do I say goodbye now, or wait until I am sure? Do I let my daughter see me like this, or protect her from it?

These are not behavioral choices in the way "do I take the pill" is a behavioral choice. They are orientations. They do not get decided once. They get revisited every day, every visit, every phone call at 2 a.m. when the pain is bad and the world feels impossible.

Treating existential ambivalence as if it were behavioral is one of the most common mistakes in end of life communication. It shows up when the clinician says "let's make a decision about your goals of care today" and the patient goes quiet. It shows up when the social worker tries to "help the family come to consensus" about hospice. It shows up when the physician offers a plan that sounds clean and the family leaves the meeting with all the feelings they had walked in with plus new guilt about not agreeing cleanly.

A patient with existential ambivalence does not need you to help them decide. They need you to help them see what they are carrying and name it accurately. Once that happens, sometimes a decision follows. Sometimes it does not. Either way, the patient is less alone with what they feel, which is often the most therapeutic thing you can offer.

3.3 Sustain Talk At End Of Life

In MI, the patient's own language divides into two categories. **Change talk** is any statement that moves toward the change under consideration. **Sustain talk** is any statement that moves away from it. In classical MI, you are listening for change talk and gently amplifying it, because the more change talk a patient speaks, the more likely they are to change.

At end of life, this map needs redrawing. What counts as change? If the patient is dying and refusing hospice, is the "change" enrolling in hospice? Or is the change learning to accept what is happening, whatever form that takes? The behavior lens does not quite fit.

Here is a more useful reframe. Sustain talk at end of life is usually about protecting something. The patient who says "I don't want hospice" is often protecting hope, identity, family relationships, or the sense that they are still fighting. The daughter who says "I can't stop feeding her" is protecting the bond she has had with her mother for her whole life. These are not obstacles to overcome. They are the things that make the patient who they are.

When you treat sustain talk as resistance to be overcome, two bad things happen. First, the patient feels you are trying to take away something that matters to them, and they dig in harder. Second, you miss the chance to hear what they are actually protecting, which is usually the door to the whole conversation.

Reflecting sustain talk sounds counterintuitive. It feels like you are agreeing with the thing you are trying to move. You are not. You are showing the patient you understand what is underneath the words. When they feel understood, they often move on their own.

Consider a wife who says "I can't stop giving him the morphine, I know he needs it but I feel like I am killing him." The rescue move is to reassure: "You are not killing him, the morphine does not cause death." The MI move is to reflect what is underneath: "Giving him that medicine feels like a betrayal of the vows you made." Nine times out of ten, that second move leads to her talking about what she is actually wrestling with, which is the helplessness of watching him die, not a misunderstanding about pharmacology.

3.4 Change Talk As Acceptance

Change talk at end of life often does not sound like "I am going to do X." It sounds like small openings. "I guess I know this is not going to get better." "Maybe it is time." "I don't want her to suffer like my dad did." "I keep thinking I should tell the kids."

These are fragile statements. They are the patient or family member testing out a thought that was too heavy to say a week ago. Your response to them matters enormously. If you pounce on the opening and try to convert it into a decision, the speaker often retreats. "Oh, so you want to enroll in hospice today?" can shut down the very opening you just heard.

The MI response is to receive the change talk and invite more. "You are starting to see that it is not going to get better. What else is on your mind about that?" This does two things. It acknowledges what they said. And it signals that you are a safe place to keep thinking out loud.

Most end of life change talk is not about a behavior. It is about an internal shift toward accepting a reality the person has been holding at arm's length. Your job is to be the place where that shift can happen without judgment, without pushing, without hurry.

One more point. Change talk in this setting is often followed immediately by sustain talk. The family member who said "I think she would want to be comfortable" will say, ninety seconds later, "but I can't just let her go." Both are real. Both belong in the conversation. A clinician who hears the first and tries to pin it down will lose the second, which is the one that still has work to do.

3.5 A Real Example

Meet David. He was a 54 year old man with amyotrophic lateral sclerosis, about fourteen months from diagnosis, still living at home with his wife Fatima. His speech had started to fail. His hospice nurse, Aisha, was visiting twice a week.

On one visit, David used his letter board to spell out: "I want to die before I can't breathe on my own."

Aisha had been trained on what to say and not say about physician assisted dying in her state. She had a protocol in her head. She did not reach for it. She asked him what he meant.

He spelled: "I don't want Fatima to watch that."

Aisha said, "You are thinking about protecting her."

He spelled: "Yes. But I don't want to leave yet either."

She said, "You want to protect her and you also are not ready to go."

He looked at her for a long time. Then he slowly spelled: "Both true. I don't know what to do with that."

She said, "You don't have to know tonight."

They sat in silence for maybe ten minutes. When Fatima came back into the room with tea, David spelled one word: "Tired."

Aisha left the visit thinking she had done very little. Three weeks later, David asked her to help him write down what he wanted his last weeks to look like. He did not pick a date. He did not make a plan. He named the things that mattered to him, and the things he wanted Fatima to know, and the ways he wanted to be treated when he could no longer speak at all. That document shaped every subsequent decision his family made.

What this means for you: David's ambivalence was not a puzzle to solve. It was two honest truths he was carrying at the same time. Aisha's refusal to pick one of them for him, and her willingness to name both out loud, gave him the room to find his own way forward. That forward did not look like a decision. It looked like clarity.

3.6 Another Real Example

Meet James. He was a 29 year old ICU nurse in Houston who had been redeployed to a palliative care consult service after two years of bedside ICU work. He was bright, confident, and new to end of life conversations outside of code situations.

On his third week, he was with a family whose matriarch was in the final days of congestive heart failure. The oldest son, Omar, had been the one making decisions. Omar had agreed to hospice transfer but kept saying "I just keep thinking maybe we should try the diuretic one more time."

James, trained to believe ambivalence was to be resolved, started reviewing the medical rationale for stopping the diuretic. He explained fluid dynamics. He explained comfort medications. He explained the signs of imminent death. Omar nodded and kept saying "I know, I know." At the end of the meeting, Omar said, "Let me think about it," and left.

James's preceptor pulled him aside afterward. She asked him what he thought Omar had been saying. James said, "He was not accepting the plan. I was trying to help him accept it."

The preceptor said, "What if he was telling you he wasn't done yet. Not with the diuretic. With being her son. With being the one who made decisions. With her. What if the 'one more time' wasn't about fluid."

James went back the next morning. He found Omar in the family lounge. He said, "Tell me about your mother."

Omar talked for forty minutes. About growing up. About her cooking. About how she had always been the one who knew what to do and he had never been the one in charge until now. By the end he said, "I don't actually want the diuretic. I just want her back."

James said, "Yes."

Omar started planning her last days. The diuretic did not come up again.

What this means for you: Ambivalence is almost never about the medical thing it appears to be about. When a family member keeps circling back to a clinical decision that seems settled, the ambivalence is usually about something deeper that they have not been able to name. Your job is not to win the medical argument. It is to let them find the thing underneath.

3.7 Why Pushing Backfires

Here is the most important sentence in this chapter: when you push against sustain talk, it gets louder.

This is not a metaphor. It is a repeatedly observed pattern in communication research. When a clinician argues the case for a change, the patient generates more sustain talk in response. The more the clinician pushes, the more the patient defends. By the end of the conversation, the patient has talked themselves more deeply into the sustain position than they were in at the start (Miller and Rose, 2013; Apodaca and Longabaugh, 2009).

This is the **righting reflex**, and it is one of the most important things Miller and Rollnick named. It is the automatic urge the clinician has to correct, argue, persuade, or convince when they see a patient heading toward a decision they believe is wrong. The reflex feels helpful. It is the opposite of helpful.

The math is simple. Every time you make the case for hospice to a resistant patient, you force them to generate reasons against hospice to defend their autonomy. They are listening to themselves say "I don't need hospice" more than they are listening to you say "you do need hospice." Whose voice do they trust more in their own head? Theirs. So you have just helped them talk themselves out of the thing you wanted.

This is counterintuitive. It violates everything the clinician was trained to do, which is to provide information, explain clearly, and guide patients toward medically appropriate care. The MI finding is not that explanation and guidance are wrong. It is that they are ineffective when the patient is in an ambivalent state, and the most effective intervention is to help them hear their own change talk.

The practical move is called **rolling with resistance**. When you hear sustain talk, you do not push back. You reflect it, sometimes amplify it slightly, and let the patient hear themselves. Often the patient follows up with change talk on their own. When they do, you reflect that too. The patient has now argued both sides out loud, and has usually moved further toward a decision than any amount of persuasion would have produced.

This is not a trick. It is not manipulation. It only works when you are genuinely curious about what they think. If you are using the technique to get them to a predetermined outcome, the patient will smell it, and the whole thing collapses. Which is why the spirit of MI has to come first.

3.8 When It Does Not Work

The most common place this breaks down is when the patient's ambivalence is not really ambivalence at all, but a cover for something else. A patient who keeps saying "maybe I should try more chemo" may not be ambivalent about hospice. They may be terrified, or they may be trying to please a family member who is not in the room, or they may have a specific fear (pain, abandonment, becoming a burden) that they have not been able to say out loud.

When you reflect what looks like ambivalence and the patient does not move, that is usually a sign that the real issue has not surfaced. Three things to try:

1. Ask a gentle open question about what they are worried about. Not about the decision, about what is underneath it. "What are you most afraid of right now?" is a hard question to ask and often the one that unlocks the room. 2. Check for the unspoken relative. "Who else is part of this decision for you?" often surfaces that they are not really wrestling with their own preference, they are wrestling with what a spouse or child or pastor will think. 3. Name the specific fear you suspect. "Some patients in your situation are afraid that hospice means they will be forgotten by their doctor. Is that something on your mind?" Offering a possibility lets the patient confirm or deny without having to originate the admission.

If after all this the conversation still does not move, it is often fine to let it sit. You do not have to resolve anything today. The patient may need to live with what you reflected for a week before they are ready to talk again. The hospice is still going to be there. So are you.

3.9 Before You Move On

Ambivalence at end of life is not a problem to fix. It is the normal state of people facing death. It is almost always existential rather than behavioral, meaning both sides of what the patient feels are permanently true rather than resolvable. Trying to resolve it through argument or explanation triggers the righting reflex, which makes the patient defend their position more strongly and move further from the change you hoped for.

The move instead is to treat sustain talk as information about what the patient is protecting, and to reflect it without pushing. Change talk in this setting often looks like small openings toward acceptance rather than toward a behavior. When you hear these openings, you receive them and invite more, rather than converting them into decisions. The same conversation often contains both sustain and change talk, sometimes in the same sentence, and both belong.

The most important move you will make in this book starts here: refusing the urge to fix what is not broken. Ambivalence is the patient's way of telling you what they are living with. Your job is to help them carry it, not to lift it off them. The next chapter turns to a related tension, the one between the directive roots of MI and the non directive work that much of end of life care requires.

Chapter 4: When To Guide Or Follow

Dr. Yuki Tanaka had practiced palliative medicine for twelve years. She was known among the oncology staff as the person you called when a family was "stuck." She had a reputation for patience, for not pushing families into decisions, for letting them arrive at clarity on their own terms. She was good at the work.

On a Thursday morning, she walked into a family meeting she had been dreading. The patient was a 34 year old woman named Layla with metastatic ovarian cancer. She had two young children, a husband named Marcus, and a mother who had flown in from out of state. Layla had been in the medical ICU for eleven days. She was intubated, sedated, on three pressors. Her oncologist had recommended a fourth line chemotherapy agent that had a 3 percent response rate in her specific disease state and a serious side effect profile that would likely accelerate her death.

The family wanted to try the chemo.

Yuki sat down. She listened to the oncologist explain. She listened to the mother describe her daughter's strength. She listened to Marcus say they just wanted to give her a chance. Every MI instinct in her body said "reflect, evoke, hold space." And she knew, in her bones, that she could not do only that in this meeting.

The chemo was not a reasonable option. It had near zero probability of helping Layla and near certainty of harming her. The family was not ambivalent about it, they were sure they wanted it. A non directive response would leave them with a treatment plan that would cause their loved one to die in more suffering than she was already in.

Yuki did something that felt uncomfortable but necessary. She said, "I have to tell you something, and I want to say it gently, but I want to say it clearly. The treatment being discussed is very unlikely to help Layla and is likely to make her last days harder. I want to talk with you about why that is, and then I want to hear what you think."

The mother cried. Marcus looked at the floor. After a long silence, Marcus said, "So what are you telling us we should do?"

And then Yuki did something that felt like MI again. She said, "I am not telling you what to do. I am telling you what the medicine can and cannot do. What to do with that information is still yours. But I did not want you to make this decision thinking the treatment was something it is not."

That conversation held the two poles of this chapter. There are moments in palliative care when you have to be directive, moments when the patient or family deserves your clinical judgment stated plainly. There are moments when you must not be directive, when evoking their values is the only ethical move. Learning when each applies is one of the hardest judgment calls in this field. It cannot be reduced to a rule, but it can be practiced and it can be learned.

4.1 The Original MI Target

When Miller and Rollnick first described motivational interviewing in the early 1980s, they had a specific target in mind: a behavior the client was ambivalent about, which the clinician had a reasonable opinion about. Alcohol use. Drug use. Medication adherence. Smoking. In these settings, the clinician genuinely hopes for a specific outcome, and MI was designed to evoke the client's own motivation for that outcome without coercion.

This is classical MI, sometimes called **directive MI**. The word "directive" here has a specific meaning. It does not mean the clinician is bossy, argumentative, or heavy handed. It means the clinician has a goal in mind and is evoking in that direction. They are not trying to be neutral. They are trying to help the client find their own reasons for the change the clinician believes would be good for them.

The skills are the same as in any MI encounter: open questions, reflections, summaries, eliciting change talk. The difference is directional. In directive MI, the clinician amplifies change talk toward the target behavior and does not amplify sustain talk. Over time, the patient hears themselves argue in favor of change more than against it, and behavior tends to follow.

This framework maps onto many parts of palliative care practice. Medication adherence is a common target: a patient not taking their scheduled morphine is a patient whose pain is not controlled, and the clinician has a reasonable goal of helping them take the medication as prescribed. Completion of advance directives is another target: a patient without an appointed healthcare proxy is at risk, and the clinician has a reasonable goal of helping them appoint one. Smoking in the setting of advanced COPD is another.

In these situations, directive MI is appropriate. You are not neutral. You have a position. Your job is to help the patient find their own way to that position without coercion.

4.2 The Palliative Target

Much of palliative care, though, does not have a clean behavioral target. Consider the patient with metastatic cancer deciding how to spend their last months. Consider the family deciding about withdrawing ventilation. Consider the dementia patient's son deciding if she should be resuscitated.

What is the "correct" outcome in these cases? There usually is not one. There are outcomes that align with the patient's values and outcomes that do not. But the clinician is often not in a position to say which is which, because the values are the patient's and the clinician does not hold them.

This is **non directive MI**, sometimes called **MI with equipoise**. In this frame, the clinician is genuinely neutral about which direction the patient moves, because the clinician believes either direction could be consistent with the patient's values. The skills are the same. The amplification pattern is different. Rather than amplifying change talk toward a predetermined target, the clinician amplifies whatever talk seems to reveal the patient's own values, and reflects both sides of ambivalence without weighting one.

Black and Helgason (2018) analyzed this carefully. They noted that non directive MI in end of life settings requires more skill than directive MI, not less. Metaphorically, non directive MI is a tightrope walk. Precise balance is needed. The clinician who tilts subtly toward their own preferred outcome, even without meaning to, can nudge the patient in a direction that is not theirs.

The palliative care target is usually not a behavior. It is **values concordance**: the alignment of the care plan with what actually matters to the patient and family. You do not know in advance what that plan looks like. You do not get to have a preference. Your job is to help the patient or family articulate what they want their last weeks to contain, and then you help them get as close to that as the medical reality allows.

4.3 When Directive MI Fits

There are times in end of life care when directive MI is clearly the right posture. The clearest cases involve **concrete behaviors that affect comfort and safety** where the clinician has a reasonable clinical opinion and the patient's values do not obviously point the other way.

Taking prescribed opioids for pain control is the archetypal case. A patient whose pain is undermedicated is a patient who is suffering, and the clinician has a responsibility to help them use their medications effectively. Most patients who underuse opioids are not rejecting pain control philosophically; they are operating on fears about addiction, tolerance, or appearing weak. These fears respond beautifully to MI, but the MI is directed toward better adherence, not neutral with respect to the outcome. The same applies to taking anti emetics, using a commode instead of trying to walk to the bathroom, or letting a caregiver help with bathing.

Completing advance care planning documents fits here too. Most patients benefit from appointing a healthcare proxy and having some documented preferences. The clinician's goal is not to dictate what those preferences should be, but to help the patient complete the documents at all. That is directive in the procedural sense, neutral in the content sense.

Home safety is another case. A fall in a patient with end stage disease often leads to hospitalization, pain, and a compressed timeline. Helping the family install a shower bar or use a walker is something the clinician legitimately advocates for.

In all of these cases, the directive move follows the same MI structure. You ask open questions about the patient's own concerns. You reflect what you hear. You affirm what is working. You offer your clinical judgment when invited, and sometimes when not invited. But you amplify in the direction you believe serves the patient's welfare, because you have a reasoned clinical opinion about what that welfare looks like and the patient has not given you reason to think their values point elsewhere.

4.4 When Non Directive Fits

The cases that require non directive MI are the ones where the patient's values, not your clinical judgment, have to determine the answer. The paradigm examples are:

The timing of hospice enrollment. Some patients will enroll the day they become eligible; others will wait until their last week. Both can be consistent with different value systems. Your job is not to get them enrolled earlier, it is to help them clarify what they want.

The level of aggressiveness of care. Some patients want every available treatment that offers any chance, even a small one. Others want to stop sooner. Neither is right or wrong.

The location of death. Home, hospice house, hospital. Each carries different meanings for different families. You do not know which one fits.

What and how to tell family members. Some patients want full disclosure to everyone. Others want to protect their children from knowing until the end. Neither is universally right.

Continued artificial nutrition and hydration in a patient nearing death. The medical data suggests these usually do not help and can cause discomfort. The symbolic meaning for some families is such that stopping is experienced as abandonment. A non directive posture says: I will tell you what the evidence shows and what symptoms to expect either way, and then I will help you make the choice that fits your family's meaning.

In these situations, if you push, you are imposing your own values on a decision that is not yours. Even subtle pushing (through which change talk you reflect, which sustain talk you let pass, which pauses you fill) can tilt the outcome. The discipline of non directive MI is recognizing these situations and staying in equipoise even when you have a personal preference.

Here is a practical test. Before you walk into the conversation, ask yourself: "If the patient makes choice A, will I be relieved, and if they make choice B, will I be disappointed?" If the answer is yes, you are not in equipoise, and you need to examine why. Sometimes the examination reveals you have a clinical reason to prefer A (in which case you may need to shift to directive MI transparently and name your position). Sometimes it reveals a personal preference that does not actually belong in the room (in which case you need to set it aside).

4.5 A Real Example

Meet Gemma. She was a palliative care nurse practitioner working in a small rural hospital in Oregon. Her patient was a 78 year old widower named Hassan with advanced heart failure. He had been offered an LVAD, a device that could have extended his life by a year or more but required ongoing medical management and lifestyle changes. His cardiologist strongly recommended it. His two children strongly recommended it. Hassan was not sure.

When Gemma met with Hassan alone, he said, "Everyone wants me to do this. My daughter cries. My son keeps showing me articles. The cardiologist practically had it booked."

Gemma asked, "What do you think?"

Hassan was quiet for a long time. He said, "I don't want to be a patient for a year. I have been a patient for two years. I wanted to be a grandfather."

Gemma said, "The LVAD feels like more patient life, and you are done with patient life."

He said, "Yes. But I also do not want to hurt them."

This was not a case for directive MI. Gemma had no clinical or ethical position that Hassan should get the LVAD over declining it. Both choices were legitimate. Her job was to help him find his own clarity, not to tilt him toward either.

She did not argue for the LVAD. She did not argue against it. She asked what he imagined the next year looking like with the device. She asked what he imagined the next months looking like without it. She reflected what she heard. She did not summarize in a direction. She let both pictures sit in the room.

At the end of the visit, Hassan said, "I think I need to say no, and I think I need to tell the kids myself." Gemma helped him plan that conversation. She did not plan the outcome. She planned the approach.

What this means for you: Non directive MI is not passive. Gemma asked many questions, offered many reflections, helped Hassan structure his own thinking. The non directive part was that she did not tilt toward either option. She trusted Hassan to find his answer, because the answer was his and only his to find.

4.6 Another Real Example

Meet Miguel again, the oncologist from Chapter 1.0. Six months after the Tanaka conversation, he had been working on his MI skills. He had read Pollak and Arnold. He had attended a weekend training. He was trying to practice.

He had a new patient, Mr. Rivera, a 61 year old man with advanced prostate cancer. Mr. Rivera was refusing to take his prescribed oxycodone for bone pain. He said he was fine. He was not fine. His grimacing during the physical exam, his weight loss, and his wife's reports all suggested his pain was poorly controlled.

Miguel had a decision to make. Was this a case for non directive MI, where he should evoke Mr. Rivera's own values about pain control and let him decide? Or was this a case for directive MI, where he should amplify change talk toward taking the medication?

Miguel decided it was directive. The clinical opinion was clear: Mr. Rivera's pain was undermedicated, his quality of life was suffering, and there was no values based reason to suspect he preferred pain to pain control. The ambivalence was operating on fear, not on values.

But Miguel did not lecture. He asked what worried Mr. Rivera about taking the oxycodone. Mr. Rivera talked about his nephew who had become addicted to opioids after a back surgery. Miguel reflected that fear. He affirmed how seriously Mr. Rivera was taking his family history. Then he said, "I want to share some information with you that might change how you see this. Is that okay?"

Mr. Rivera said yes. Miguel explained how opioid use in advanced cancer differs from the nephew's situation. He explained that addiction is measured in less than one percent of cancer patients using opioids appropriately. He asked what Mr. Rivera thought now that he had heard that.

Mr. Rivera said, "Maybe I could try a lower dose."

Miguel did not argue for a higher dose. He said, "That is a reasonable place to start." Then he scheduled a follow up in a week.

What this means for you: Directive MI in this setting does not mean pushing. It means you have a clinical position, you share it transparently, you elicit and respect the patient's concerns, you provide information with permission, and you amplify the change talk that emerges. The patient still makes the decision. You just do not pretend to be neutral when you are not.

4.7 Equipoise As Daily Practice

The hardest part of this chapter is not deciding which posture to adopt in a given moment. The hardest part is being honest with yourself about which posture you are actually in.

Most clinicians who believe they are using non directive MI are actually tilting subtly toward their preferred outcome. They do not realize it. They reflect change talk toward that outcome with slightly more warmth than sustain talk away from it. They fill silences after statements they agree with and hold silence longer after statements they do not. They follow up with questions in the direction they want. Every single one of these moves is small. Together, they steer.

The discipline of **equipoise** is the daily practice of catching yourself in these tilts. It is asking, before each conversation, "what outcome would I prefer here, and am I willing to genuinely hold that preference aside." It is debriefing after hard conversations with a trusted colleague and asking, "did I stay neutral, or did I push." It is noticing when you feel relieved at a patient's decision and asking what that relief is telling you about what you were secretly hoping for.

None of this means you cannot have opinions. You can and should. The discipline is to know when your opinion belongs in the room and when it does not. Directive MI is a legitimate and sometimes essential practice, but it requires you to declare your direction transparently, not to smuggle it in.

A team of palliative clinicians in a large academic center developed a simple internal check. Before entering any family meeting, each clinician writes down, on an index card, what outcome they hope for and why. Then they show the card to a colleague. The colleague asks two questions. "Is that outcome based on clinical evidence that points clearly in one direction, or on your personal comfort?" And, "If the family picks something else, will you be able to support them without reservation?" The exercise takes ninety seconds. It changes what happens in the meeting.

Equipoise is not neutrality of feeling. You will have feelings. Equipoise is neutrality of pressure. You keep the room open for the patient's answer even when you desperately want a particular one. That is the craft. It is harder than any of the skills you have learned in this book so far, and it is the one that most separates experienced MI practitioners in palliative care from beginners.

4.8 When It Does Not Work

The most common place this breaks down is that the clinician cannot tell which mode to be in. They waver. They are directive for a few minutes, then non directive, then directive again. The patient experiences this as inconsistency and stops trusting either posture.

If you notice yourself wavering mid conversation, it is usually because the situation is genuinely ambiguous. Some decisions have one element that deserves directive input (like safety or symptom control) and another element that deserves non directive input (like where the patient wants to be). Pretending these are one decision makes the conversation muddled.

Three things to try:

1. Separate the parts of the decision out loud. "There is a medical part here where I want to share my clinical opinion, and there is a values part here where I am going to ask what matters to you. Can we talk about each separately?" This lets you be directive about what is medical and non directive about what is personal. 2. If you catch yourself pushing, stop and name it. "I notice I have been leaning toward a particular answer. Let me step back and ask what you actually think." Transparency rebuilds trust faster than pretending it did not happen. 3. When you are not sure which mode fits, default to non directive first. Start with open questions about their values. If, after you have heard them, you believe a directive input is needed, you can transition. Starting directive and retreating to non directive is much harder than the reverse.

If you find you cannot hold equipoise on a particular case, that is useful information. Sometimes it means you need to hand the conversation to a colleague who does not carry your particular attachment. There is no shame in that. Recognizing your limits is part of the work.

4.9 Pulling It Together

Motivational interviewing was built as a directive method for helping ambivalent clients move toward a change their clinician had a reasoned opinion about. Much of palliative care practice uses MI that way: medication adherence, advance directives, home safety.

These are cases where you have a clinical position and you use MI skills to help the patient find their own path to it.

A significant portion of palliative care, though, requires non directive MI. The timing of hospice enrollment, the aggressiveness of care, the meanings of artificial nutrition, the telling of children, the choice of location of death. These are values decisions where the clinician is not in a position to declare a correct answer. The skill is to stay in equipoise, to genuinely hold both directions as legitimate, and to help the patient or family find their own clarity without tilting.

The honest truth is that most clinicians believe they do non directive MI better than they actually do. Small tilts (a warmer reflection here, a filled silence there) accumulate and steer the outcome. The discipline of equipoise is daily, unglamorous, and mostly invisible. It is also the difference between practice that respects the patient's autonomy and practice that quietly overrides it.

With the foundations of Part I now in place, the rest of the book moves into specific skills and situations. Chapter 5.0 begins with the first of the four OARS skills: the open question, adapted for the unique pressures of end of life conversations.

PART II: THE CORE SKILLS

50

Motivational Interviewing for Hospice and Palliative Care

Chapter 5: Open Questions That Open Hearts

Version one. Tuesday, 10:42 a.m., a hospital room on the palliative care floor. Dr. Ravi Chandra, three years out of fellowship, sat beside Mrs. Kowalski's bed. Her metastatic pancreatic cancer had progressed despite three lines of treatment. He had fifteen minutes before his next consult.

"Are you in pain today?" he asked. "A little."

"Are you sleeping okay?" "Not really."

"Is the nausea better with the new medication?" "I guess."

"Do you have questions about what comes next?" She shook her head.

Ravi left the room with the basic signs noted, symptoms logged, and the same chart he had walked in with. Mrs. Kowalski watched the door close behind him and turned her face to the window.

Version two. Same room, same patient, same fifteen minutes. Different opening.

"Mrs. Kowalski, how has this week been for you?"

She took a long breath. "It has been strange. My son came from Chicago."

"Tell me about that visit."

She talked for nine minutes. About her son's three kids. About the way he cried when he saw her thin. About the fact that she had not told him yet that she did not want any more chemotherapy and she did not know how to bring it up. She wiped her eyes once. Ravi did not interrupt.

When she finished, he said, "It sounds like there is something you want to tell him that you have not been able to find the words for."

She said, "Yes. I need to tell him. But I don't know how."

The rest of the visit was not about symptoms. It was about how to have the conversation she had been carrying alone for three weeks. By the time Ravi left, she had a plan. She also had a different relationship with him than the one she had with version one Ravi, who she would never quite trust again.

This chapter is about the difference between those two visits. You will learn why clinicians default to closed questions when the pressure is on, what open questions do that closed questions cannot, and how to use open questions in a first visit, under time pressure, and when surfacing values. You will also get specific scripts you can use on your next shift. Nothing fancy. Just the few questions that change what happens in the room.

5.1 Why Closed Questions Dominate

An **open question** is a question that invites a broad answer and cannot be answered with a single word. "How has this week been?" is open. A **closed question** can be answered yes, no, or with a number. "Are you in pain?" is closed. Both have their place. The problem is that clinicians under stress default to closed, and end of life conversations need open.

Several pressures push you toward closed questions. Time is the first one. Closed questions produce fast answers, and when you have four consults left before lunch, fast feels safe. The second pressure is anxiety about the answer. Closed questions let you control what the patient is allowed to tell you. If you only ask "are you sleeping," you will never hear about the nightmares. You will never hear about the fear that is keeping the nightmares alive. The third pressure is training. You were taught to take a review of systems, which is a closed question cascade. It is efficient for ruling out appendicitis. It is useless for finding out what a dying person is carrying.

The research is clear. Studies of oncologist patient visits have found that most clinician questions in serious illness conversations are closed, and that clinicians who use more open questions build rapport faster and elicit more information about what matters to patients (Pollak et al., 2011). In MI fidelity scoring, one of the behaviors coded is the ratio of open to closed questions (Moyers et al., 2016). Experienced MI clinicians ask more open questions than closed ones. Novices reverse the ratio, which is why their sessions feel like interviews and not like conversations.

The fix is not to abandon closed questions. You still need to know the pain score and the bowel pattern. The fix is to shift your opening. Start a visit with an open question. Use the first minute or two to actually find out what is going on. Then use closed questions later to nail down the specifics. Open first, closed after. That sequence alone will change what your visits feel like.

5.2 Open Questions For First Visits

The first visit sets the tone for every visit that follows. If your opening question signals "I am here to take a checklist," the patient will give you their checklist self. If it signals "I am here to learn about you," you will get something different.

The best first visit opener in palliative care is almost always a variant of "tell me about yourself." It sounds too simple to work. It works because nobody in the medical system has asked the patient that in years.

Try one of these at your next first visit:

"Before we get into the medical stuff, tell me a little about who you are."

"What should I know about you as a person, not just a patient?"

"What were you doing before all of this started?"

"When you are not here in this room, what does your life look like?"

The answers you get will be short at first. Patients are used to being asked about their bodies. They are not used to being asked about themselves. Give them time. A beat of silence after an open question is not a failure, it is a gift. The patient is deciding how much to tell you. What they decide depends partly on what you do with that silence.

Another strong first visit move is to ask about the illness in the patient's own words rather than your words. "What have you been told about your illness?" is a powerful open question because it reveals two things at once: what the patient understands and what they are willing to say out loud. You would be surprised how often a patient's explanation of their disease does not match the chart. You would also be surprised how often they have never actually said the word "cancer" or "failing" out loud. Giving them the space to try that sentence with you is often the first therapeutic thing that happens in your relationship.

A third move is to ask about support. "Who in your life knows what is happening?" tells you who the patient considers family and who they are hiding from. "Who is taking care of you?" tells you about the caregiver system you are walking into. These questions feel like small talk. They are not. They are assessment.

5.3 Open Questions When Time Is Short

Most palliative and hospice clinicians will tell you they do not have time for open questions. The opposite is true. Open questions save time. Closed questions feel efficient because each one is brief, but a string of closed questions rarely produces useful information. You can spend ten minutes asking closed questions and walk out knowing almost nothing about the patient. You can spend three minutes on one good open question and walk out with what you actually came for.

The efficiency comes from what the open question triggers. A patient who answers "how has this week been" will usually volunteer the information you were going to ask about anyway, plus several things you did not know to ask. The nausea comes up. The sleep issue comes up. The fight with the daughter comes up. You did not have to interview your way to any of it.

Here are three open questions that work even when you have seven minutes:

"What has been on your mind this week?"

"What is the hardest part right now?"

"What do you wish the team understood about what you are going through?"

The third one is especially powerful because it positions the patient as the expert on their own situation and asks for their teaching. Most patients have never been asked that question in any clinical encounter. Their answer often reveals the one thing that, once addressed, makes every subsequent visit easier.

One caution. When you ask a time efficient open question, you have to be willing to listen to the answer. If you ask "what has been on your mind" and then interrupt thirty seconds in because you need to chart the bowel movement, you have done worse than if you had not asked at all. Open questions require a minute of uninterrupted listening. If you cannot give that minute today, use closed questions today and come back with the open one tomorrow.

5.4 A Real Example

Meet Gemma. She was a home hospice nurse who had been on her case with Mr. Bellamy for two weeks. He had advanced Parkinson's disease with early dementia. His daughter Layla was the primary caregiver. Gemma had been worried about Layla. She looked exhausted at every visit.

On her fourth visit, Gemma made a deliberate choice. Instead of asking her usual rounds of closed questions about medication compliance and bowel movements, she sat down at the kitchen table with Layla and said, "How are you holding up, really?"

Layla cried for forty seconds without saying anything. Then she said, "I am not sleeping. My brother is in Arizona and he calls once a week to second guess everything. My kids are asking when grandpa is going to die and I don't know what to tell them. And I am starting to resent my dad, which makes me feel like the worst daughter in the world."

Gemma did not start problem solving. She said, "Tell me more about the resentment."

Layla did. For ten minutes. It turned out the resentment was really grief. She was mourning the father he used to be while caring for the father he had become. She had not had anyone to say that to.

Gemma left that day having done exactly zero of the teaching points she had on her list. She had also done the single most useful thing anyone had done for Layla in six months. At her next visit, Layla was a different caregiver, because she had been seen once.

What this means for you: An open question is not a technique. It is an act of trust. You trust the answer will tell you what you actually need to know. Gemma was not trying to surface the resentment. She had no agenda. She was asking an open question and listening to what came out. That is the difference between doing an open question and being in an open posture.

5.5 Questions That Surface Values

There is a specific category of open question that surfaces what matters most to a patient. These are the questions that belong in goals of care conversations, advance care planning discussions, and any moment when the team needs to know what a patient is living for.

The classic MI version is the **values question**. "What is most important to you in the life you have right now?" It sounds abstract. In practice, patients answer it concretely. They say things like "being home for my granddaughter's first birthday" or "not being a burden on my wife" or "getting to fish one more time." Those answers are more useful than any checklist.

Other values surfacing questions include:

"What would a good day look like for you right now?"

"When you imagine the next few months, what do you hope for?"

"When you imagine the next few months, what do you worry about?"

"If things do not go the way we hope, what matters most to you about how they do go?"

"What would it look like for your family to know they did right by you?"

These questions are adapted from several frameworks, including the Serious Illness Conversation Guide developed by Ariadne Labs (Bernacki and Block, 2014). That guide has been used in more than thirteen thousand clinicians' training, and a cluster randomized trial in outpatient oncology found that patients whose clinicians used it reported less anxiety and depression than those who received usual care (Bernacki et al., 2019). The magic of the guide is not in the specific words. It is in the commitment to open, values focused questions over closed, fact focused ones.

One warning. These questions can unearth powerful emotion. A patient who has been holding it together for months may crack open when you ask what they are hoping for. Be ready to sit with what comes out. If you ask the question and then look uncomfortable when they cry, you have taught them not to trust you with the next hard thing.

5.6 Another Real Example

Meet James. He was an internist who had just started moonlighting at a local hospice. He had been a hospitalist for fourteen years. He was used to efficient interviews. His attending at the hospice, a palliative medicine doc named Fatima, had asked him to try opening his visits with a single value question instead of a review of symptoms.

On his first try, he walked into Mr. Okafor's room and said, "Mr. Okafor, what is most important to you right now?"

Mr. Okafor stared at him for a long time. Then he said, "I want to live long enough to watch my son graduate."

James had not known the son was graduating. He had not known there was a son. His chart said "widower, no local family."

"Tell me about your son."

Twenty minutes later, James had learned that the son had been estranged for eleven years, had reconnected two months before the diagnosis, and was flying in for graduation in three weeks. Mr. Okafor wanted to be there. The medical team had been planning to admit him for aggressive symptom management that would have prevented travel. Nobody had asked.

James changed the plan. The symptom management was reorganized around the graduation. Mr. Okafor made the trip. He died two weeks after he came back. His son came for the funeral.

What this means for you: Values questions can reorganize a care plan in a way that no amount of symptom management can. The patient's answer may contradict what was already written in the chart. When it does, the patient's answer wins. Your job is not to deliver the plan, it is to build the plan around what they just told you matters.

5.7 Scripts You Can Memorize

This section gives you specific questions to take into your next shift. Pick two or three. Write them on an index card. Use them for a week. Then come back for two more.

For the opening of any visit:

"How has this week been for you?"

"What has been on your mind since I saw you last?"

"What would be most helpful for us to talk about today?"

For first visits:

"Before we talk about your medical care, tell me a little about who you are."

"What have you been told about your illness?"

"Who in your life knows what is happening?"

For surfacing values:

"What is most important to you right now?"

"What would a good day look like?"

"What are you hoping for?"

"What are you worrying about?"

For goals of care conversations:

"If things do not go the way we hope, what matters most to you?"

"What would you want your family to know about what you want?"

"When you think about the next few weeks, what are you picturing?"

For caregivers:

"How are you holding up, really?"

"What is the hardest part of caring for him right now?"

"What do you wish the team understood about your situation?"

For the close of a visit:

"What questions are you sitting with that we have not talked about?"

"What do you want to remember from this conversation?"

"What is the most important thing you want us to do before I see you next?"

These are not magic. They are the plain, direct questions that work because they are plain and direct. Resist the urge to dress them up. "Would you be open to sharing with me, if it is not too intrusive, some of your reflections on what you might be thinking about regarding your preferences" is not a question, it is an apology. Ask the simpler thing.

5.8 When It Does Not Work

The most common way open questions fail is that the clinician asks one and then does not wait for the answer. The patient takes a breath, starts to organize their thoughts, and the clinician fills the pause with clarification or a follow up. The answer dies before it reaches speech.

This is not impatience. It is discomfort with silence. A silence after an open question feels like a failure because you are not doing anything. You are doing something. You are making room. The patient needs a few seconds to decide how honest they want to be. If you fill those seconds, you have just answered the question for them, and their answer will be a safer, shallower version of what they would have said.

Three things to try:

1. Ask your open question. Then count to seven in your head before you say anything. Seven seconds feels like an eternity and is usually exactly the right amount of time. 2. When you feel the urge to clarify, ask yourself if you are clarifying for them or for yourself. If you are not sure, wait. 3. If the patient truly does not answer, try one gentle follow up: "Take your time." Then go back to waiting.

A second common failure is asking an open question when you do not have time for the answer. If you have three minutes left and you ask "what has been on your mind," you have just opened a door you cannot walk through. It is better to say "I have only a few minutes today. Is there one thing you want me to know before I come back Thursday?" That is a bounded open question. It respects the clock and still invites the truth.

If you try this for a month and still feel like open questions are making your visits longer, it is worth asking a colleague to observe one. Often what looks like an open question problem is actually a listening problem, and somebody else can spot it faster than you can.

5.9 The Short Answer

Clinicians under stress default to closed questions because they feel fast and controllable. They are neither. Closed questions produce a review of systems. Open questions produce a relationship. Closed questions tell you the pain score. Open questions tell you what the pain is costing the patient, which is what actually shapes the care plan.

The shift is simple and hard. Open first, closed after. Start every visit with one genuine open question. Wait seven seconds for the answer. Use the answer to decide where the conversation should go. Bring your closed questions in later, after you know what you are actually dealing with.

First visits benefit from "tell me about yourself" openers and questions about how the patient understands their illness. Short visits benefit from bounded open questions like "what is the hardest part right now." Goals of care conversations need values questions: what matters most, what are you hoping for, what are you worrying about. The Serious Illness Conversation Guide offers a structured set of these that has been tested in thousands of patients.

Keep an index card with three questions you are practicing this week. Read them before each visit. After a month of this, the questions will be in your mouth without the card. Open questions are the first of the four OARS skills. The next chapter is about the second, affirmations, and why most of what clinicians call affirmation is actually something else entirely.

Chapter 6: Affirmations Without False Comfort

Akira was a hospice CNA in her second year. She had been assigned to Mr. Delacroix's case for six weeks. His wife Ananya was the primary caregiver. Ananya was 74 years old and had been getting up three times a night to reposition her husband, who weighed 180 pounds and could no longer move himself.

One Thursday morning, Akira arrived to find Ananya crying at the kitchen table. She had tried to transfer her husband to the commode alone and he had slid to the floor. He was not hurt. She was shaken.

Akira wanted to help. She said what she had been taught to say. "Oh honey, you are doing such a great job. You are such a good wife. He is so lucky to have you."

Ananya smiled politely and wiped her eyes. She went back to the bedroom to finish his morning care. Akira felt she had done her job.

That afternoon the hospice social worker called Ananya to check in. Ananya broke down on the phone and said she could not do this anymore. She said everyone kept telling her she was doing a great job and she did not believe them and she was so tired of pretending to be okay when they said it.

Akira's affirmation had not only failed. It had reinforced Ananya's sense that nobody in the system could actually see what was happening in that house.

This chapter is about the difference between the **reassurance** Akira gave and the **affirmation** Ananya needed. You will learn why "you are doing a great job" usually lands as hollow, what a real affirmation looks like, how to affirm competence without dismissing exhaustion, and why there are moments when affirmation should wait. You will also see that affirmation, done right, is one of the most clinically powerful things you can offer a caregiver or patient in extremis.

6.1 Why "Great Job" Fails

The problem with "you are doing a great job" is that it is abstract, generic, and often delivered to silence the clinician's own discomfort rather than to serve the person receiving it. It sounds supportive. It is actually a kind of brush off.

Three things make this specific phrase fail.

First, it is unspecific. The person saying it could be saying it to anyone. It contains no evidence that the speaker has actually observed the listener doing anything. A 74 year old woman who has been lifting her husband at 3 a.m. for six weeks can smell a generic compliment from across the room. She knows you are saying what you are supposed to say.

Second, it is evaluative. The clinician is positioning themselves as the judge of how well the caregiver is doing. That might feel supportive when the grade is high. It is also a power move. The caregiver did not ask for a grade. They asked, implicitly, to be seen. A grade is not the same as being seen.

Third, it forecloses what the person might say next. If Ananya had said "I am doing a great job," Akira might have asked what was hard about it. By delivering the compliment instead of asking, Akira closed the door the caregiver had just cracked open. Ananya took the brush off gracefully because that is what she does. She did not get what she came to the kitchen table hoping to find.

A genuine affirmation has none of these features. It is specific. It is descriptive rather than evaluative. It leaves room for the person to say more.

In MI, affirmations are defined as statements that recognize a specific strength, effort, or attribute in a way that is explicitly linked to the person's behavior or characteristic (Moyers et al., 2016). In the MITI coding manual used to assess MI fidelity, "I am really proud of you" does not count as an affirmation. "It is important to you to be a good parent, just like your folks were for you" does. The difference is observable, specific content rather than generic approval.

Once you start listening for it, you will hear the difference everywhere. Most workplace "great job" comments are not affirmations. They are social lubricant. They serve the speaker more than the listener.

6.2 Specific Affirmations

Here is what Akira could have said instead.

"You learned how to use the Hoyer lift in two days. That is not something most people figure out that fast."

"You have been repositioning him every two hours for six weeks. That is harder than any nursing home shift I have ever worked."

"You noticed the pressure area on his sacrum before I did yesterday. You are paying attention to things most family members would miss."

Notice what is happening in these sentences. Each one names a specific thing Ananya did. Each one is something Akira has actually observed. None of them is a grade. None of them tells Ananya she is "good." They tell her, concretely, what she has done, and they imply that Akira has been watching closely enough to know.

This is harder than generic praise. It requires you to pay attention. It requires you to have specific things to name. It requires you to remember details from previous visits. That last part is often what separates a clinician who can affirm well from one who cannot. If you do not remember that the daughter figured out how to crush the medications into applesauce three days ago, you cannot affirm her for it today.

One trick some hospice clinicians use is to keep a mental or literal note of one concrete thing each family member has done well since the last visit. Before you walk in the door, review your note. Now you have something specific to say. This is not manipulation. It is the kind of attention that turns affirmation from social noise into a clinical intervention.

Some effective affirmations are not about what the person has done but about a quality you have observed. "You have a way of reading him that I do not have." "You stay calm when he gets agitated, and that matters." These work when they are true and when they are specific enough to the person that they could not be said to anyone else in the room.

Avoid the word "should" in affirmations. "You should be proud of yourself" places you as the authority on what they ought to feel. A real affirmation does not tell the person how to feel about themselves. It tells them something accurate and trusts them to do their own feeling.

6.3 Competence Without Denying Exhaustion

One of the trickiest moments in hospice affirmation work is when a caregiver is both competent and exhausted at the same time. Generic praise ignores the exhaustion and lands as dismissive. Straight empathy ignores the competence and can land as infantilizing. Doing both at once is the craft.

Here is the structure. Name the effort. Name the cost. Do not collapse one into the other.

"You have been running on four hours of sleep for two weeks and you are still keeping his medication schedule exactly right. That is taking something out of you."

"You caught the new symptom before anyone else did, and you are exhausted because catching things is now your full time job."

"You are doing work that nurses in the ICU get trained for years to do, and you are doing it without anyone relieving you."

Each of these recognizes competence in a specific, observable way and immediately acknowledges what that competence is costing. It does not minimize. It does not rescue. It says, accurately, what is happening.

The research on caregiver wellbeing suggests this combined acknowledgment is protective. Caregivers who feel their work is seen and named report less depression and less burnout than those who feel invisible, regardless of the intensity of the care they are providing (Washington et al., 2015). Invisibility is the poison. The work is not what burns caregivers out. The work done without anyone seeing it is what burns them out.

One more note on this. Sometimes the cost needs to be named before the competence. If a caregiver walks into the conversation obviously exhausted, leading with praise will feel tone deaf. Start with the cost. "You look like you have not slept in days." Wait. Let them tell you what is happening. Then, later in the conversation, name the competence. Order matters. Meet them where they are before you tell them what you see.

6.4 A Real Example

Meet Elena. She was a hospice chaplain in her ninth year. She had been visiting Mrs. Castellano, a 68 year old woman with advanced ALS, for four months. Mrs. Castellano's husband Miguel was the primary caregiver.

On a Tuesday in October, Elena arrived to find Miguel sitting on the porch. His wife was inside with a home health aide. Miguel looked up and said, "I think I am failing her."

Elena did not say he was doing a great job. She sat down next to him and said, "Tell me what failing looks like to you."

Miguel said he had snapped at her the night before because she kept asking him to reposition her pillow. He had apologized. She had cried. He had lain awake most of the night hating himself.

Elena said, "You have been up every two hours with her for months. You snapped at her once and you apologized immediately. That is not failing, that is being human under conditions that would break most people."

Miguel started to cry. Elena did not reach for the tissue. She waited.

When Miguel stopped, Elena said, "I have been watching you for four months. I have watched you learn to suction her trach. I have watched you make her laugh on the days she could still laugh. I have watched you stay up to sit with her because she is scared at night. You are not failing her. You are loving her through something impossible."

Miguel said, "I don't feel like I am loving her. I feel like I am surviving her."

Elena said, "Both can be true."

That conversation did not fix anything. Miguel still had four more months of care ahead of him. But something shifted. He had been seen, accurately, by someone who had been watching. He went back inside. He called Elena two days later to say he had been thinking about what she said, and it had helped him sleep.

What this means for you: A real affirmation can include contradiction. Miguel was both loving and surviving. Elena did not pick one. She held both. An affirmation that only tells the comfortable half of the truth is not an affirmation, it is reassurance. Reassurance comforts the speaker. Affirmation respects the listener.

6.5 Affirming Ambivalence

Here is a move that most clinicians never learn and that changes everything once you do: affirming the ambivalence itself.

Patients and families in palliative care are often of two minds. They want hospice and they do not. They want the morphine and they are scared of it. They want to talk about death and they want to pretend it is not happening. Most clinicians, when they encounter this doubleness, try to resolve it. That usually fails.

A different move is to name the ambivalence and respect it as a sign of thoughtfulness rather than indecision. "You are weighing two things that both matter to you. That is not you being confused, that is you being careful."

You can affirm ambivalence like this:

"You are trying to honor what your mother said she wanted and you are also a son who does not want to let her go. Those are both the right things to be feeling."

"You are considering the hospice option and you are not ready to sign anything today. That tells me you are taking this seriously."

"Part of you wants to stop the chemo and part of you does not. Both parts are yours, and neither is wrong."

This reframes ambivalence from a problem to a feature of careful thinking. Patients and families often feel that their mixed feelings are evidence of weakness or failure to decide. When a clinician names the mixed feelings as legitimate, the person relaxes. Once they relax, they can often think more clearly. Many decisions that feel stuck become unstuck, not because you pushed, but because you stopped treating the ambivalence as an obstacle.

Affirming ambivalence is one of the most distinctly MI moves in this book. You will not find it in most nursing textbooks. You will find it working in homes and in ICUs and in nursing facility conference rooms every day, in the hands of clinicians who have learned it.

6.6 Another Real Example

Meet Marcus. He was a palliative medicine physician in his sixth year. His patient was Mrs. Nakamura, a 61 year old woman with advanced lung cancer. She had been going back and forth about enrolling in hospice for three weeks. Her oncologist had asked Marcus to "help her decide."

Marcus sat with Mrs. Nakamura for thirty minutes. He did not try to help her decide. At the end of the conversation, he said, "You have been thinking about this for three weeks. You have talked to your daughter, your priest, and your sister about it. You have written down the pros and cons. You are still not sure. I want to tell you something. The fact that you are not sure is not a problem. It tells me this is a big decision and you are giving it the weight it deserves. You do not have to decide today."

Mrs. Nakamura started to cry. She said, "Everyone keeps telling me I need to decide. You are the first person who has not."

Marcus said, "I will come back next week. We can talk again then."

Three days later, Mrs. Nakamura called the office. She said she was ready to enroll in hospice. She said she had not been able to decide when she felt rushed. Once someone told her she did not have to, she figured out what she actually wanted.

What this means for you: Sometimes the most useful affirmation is of the patient's right to not be ready. Decisions about death often happen when the clinician stops pushing for them. Affirming that someone is not ready can be the thing that lets them become ready.

6.7 When Affirmation Must Wait

Not every moment is an affirmation moment. Some moments call for silence. Some call for reflection. Some call for just sitting with the person in their pain. Knowing when not to affirm is as important as knowing how.

A few situations where affirmation should wait:

When the person is in fresh grief. A daughter whose father just died does not need to be told she is doing a great job. She needs someone to sit with her. Affirmation at that moment can feel like a redirect, like you are trying to make her feel better when what she needs is to feel what she feels.

When the person has just expressed something hard. If someone says "I am so angry at my husband for leaving me to deal with this alone," affirming their caregiving is a non sequitur. It says "I am not going to respond to what you actually said, I am going to respond to what I wish you had said." Reflect the anger first. Affirmation can come later, if it is still relevant.

When the affirmation would paper over a real problem. If a caregiver is clearly overwhelmed and unsafe to continue without more support, "you are doing such a great job" is a way of avoiding the harder conversation about respite or additional resources. The kind thing is often the honest thing: "This is more than one person can do alone. Let's talk about what help we can bring in."

When you do not believe it. If you are not actually impressed by what the family member is doing, do not say you are. Faked affirmations are heard. They corrode trust faster than honest silence. If you cannot find something true to affirm, do not affirm. You can still be respectful. You can still be kind. You just do not need to manufacture praise.

6.8 When It Does Not Work

The most common way affirmation goes wrong is that it slides into reassurance without the clinician noticing. You meant to recognize specific effort. What came out of your mouth was generic comfort. The caregiver nods politely. Nothing shifts. You feel good because you said a nice thing. They feel slightly worse because they were seen at arm's length.

If you notice this happening, three things to try:

1. Before your next visit, write down one specific thing each family member did since you saw them last. Not "she is doing well." Something concrete, like "she figured out the dressing change without help on Tuesday." Bring that to the visit. 2. When you feel the urge to say "you are doing a great job," stop. Ask yourself: great at what, specifically. If you cannot finish the sentence, do not start it. 3. Watch the face of the person you affirm. A real affirmation usually produces a small shift. They exhale. They soften. They look at you for a beat longer than usual. If you see no shift, your affirmation did not land. Try again differently next time.

A second failure is affirming too early. Some caregivers are not ready to hear that they are doing well. They are holding themselves together by believing they are not doing enough. If you tell them they are doing great before they are ready to hear it, the praise can feel like pressure to stop trying harder. In those cases, start with acknowledgment of difficulty. "This is brutal work." Let that sit. The affirmation can come later, once they are ready to receive it.

6.9 Pulling It Together

Most of what clinicians call affirmation is actually reassurance, and the difference matters. Reassurance is generic, evaluative, and serves the speaker's comfort. Affirmation is specific, descriptive, and serves the listener. "You are doing a great job" is reassurance. "You noticed the pressure area before I did yesterday" is affirmation.

Good affirmations name specific, observable effort or strength. They can hold contradiction, acknowledging that someone is both loving and surviving, both competent and exhausted. They can even affirm ambivalence itself, reframing mixed feelings as evidence of careful thinking rather than failure to decide.

Affirmation is not always the right move. Fresh grief, raw emotion, and safety concerns all call for different responses. The discipline is to know when to affirm, what to affirm with specificity, and when to hold silence and reflect instead.

The next chapter is about reflection, which is the single most powerful MI skill in this setting. Reflections are what you say when words are needed but advice and affirmation are not. They are how you show someone they have been heard. They are also how an entire conversation shifts in thirty seconds, with one well placed sentence.

Chapter 7: Reflections That Do The Work

Omar was a chaplain at a community hospital in Detroit. He had been asked to join a family meeting for a 46 year old man named Kenji who was dying of complications from COVID related lung damage. The meeting had seven people in it: the patient's wife, two adult children, a brother, a sister in law, the attending physician, and the ICU nurse.

The first forty minutes were chaos. The brother wanted to transfer Kenji to another hospital. The wife wanted to stop the ventilator. The older daughter had printed out an article about a clinical trial. The younger daughter was sobbing. The attending was trying to explain that transfer was not medically feasible. Nobody was hearing anyone else. Voices kept rising.

Omar had not said anything. He was listening for the thing underneath the thing.

At minute forty three, during a pause, he said to the brother, "You love him and you are not ready to be the uncle who let him die."

The brother stopped. His face changed. He said, "Yeah. That is what this is."

The room went quiet. It was the first moment of quiet in the meeting. The wife looked at Omar. The daughters looked at each other. Something had shifted.

Over the next twenty minutes, the conversation changed. The brother stopped arguing for transfer. The wife talked about what Kenji had told her two weeks before the intubation. The daughters agreed on what their father would have wanted. The attending did not have to defend the medical picture anymore because the family was no longer fighting it.

Omar drove home that night and realized the whole shift had come from one sentence. Not a lecture. Not a persuasion. One accurate reflection of what the brother was actually saying underneath what he was saying.

This chapter is about that skill. **Reflections** are the most powerful and most underused tool in end of life communication. You will learn the difference between simple and complex reflections, how to reflect feeling in a setting where feelings are overwhelming, how to reflect both sides of ambivalence at once, and when amplified reflections are useful versus when they cross into manipulation.

7.1 Simple Reflections

A **reflection** is a statement that captures what the speaker just said or implied, offered back to them in a way that lets them hear themselves. There are two broad categories. Simple reflections stay close to what the person said. Complex reflections go deeper, capturing meaning, emotion, or implication that was not explicitly spoken.

A simple reflection might restate what the person said with slightly different words. If a patient says "I just feel so tired," a simple reflection is "you are exhausted." The statement has not added much. It has confirmed that you heard. Sometimes that is exactly what the person needs.

Simple reflections seem almost too simple to matter. They matter more than they look. In a moment of high emotion, when a caregiver is crying or a patient is scared, a simple reflection does several things at once. It slows the conversation down. It signals that you are paying attention. It prevents the cascade of advice and reassurance that most clinicians reach for. It creates a tiny space for the person to take a breath.

The common mistake with simple reflections is parroting. If a caregiver says "I am so worn out" and you say "you are so worn out" in exactly the same tone, it sounds mechanical. Good simple reflections use different words than the speaker used, or capture the same meaning in a way that shows you heard the feeling behind it.

Speaker: "I can't believe this is happening to him." Parrot: "You can't believe this is happening." Simple reflection: "This doesn't feel real."

Speaker: "I just don't know what to do." Parrot: "You don't know what to do." Simple reflection: "You are stuck."

Simple reflections are a lot like the first pitch of a warmup. They are not flashy. They establish the rhythm. In MI, the research suggests that clinicians who use reflections well have a reflection to question ratio of at least one to one, meaning they offer as many reflections as questions (Moyers et al., 2016). Most untrained clinicians ask far more questions than they reflect. Bringing up your reflection count is one of the single fastest ways to improve the quality of a conversation.

7.2 Complex Reflections

A **complex reflection** adds meaning the speaker did not explicitly say. It captures an implication, a feeling, or a value the speaker is communicating but has not named. The MITI coding manual defines a complex reflection as one where the clinician "makes a guess" at what the person is trying to communicate, going beyond what was said (Moyers et al., 2016).

Complex reflections are harder than simple ones because they require you to listen for what is underneath. They are also the single most powerful clinical move in MI. Research on MI effectiveness suggests that clinicians who use more complex reflections have better outcomes than those who mostly use simple reflections (Magill et al., 2018). The benchmark for MI proficiency is that at least 40 percent of a clinician's reflections should be complex (Moyers et al., 2016).

Here are examples of simple versus complex reflections on the same statements:

Speaker: "Everyone keeps telling me what to do." Simple: "People are giving you a lot of advice." Complex: "You are tired of being told, and you want someone to ask."

Speaker: "I don't know if I can keep doing this." Simple: "You are exhausted." Complex: "You are wondering how much longer you can hold up, and you are scared of what it means that you are wondering."

Speaker: "He is not the man I married." Simple: "He has changed a lot." Complex: "You are grieving him already, even as you are still taking care of him."

Complex reflections take risks. You are guessing at what is underneath. Sometimes you get it wrong. That is fine. When you are wrong, the person will correct you, and the correction is more valuable than a perfect guess would have been, because now the person has articulated what they actually meant. A wrong reflection that prompts a clarification is almost as useful as a right one. The only wrong kind of reflection is no reflection.

Omar's reflection in the opening ("you are not ready to be the uncle who let him die") was complex. The brother had not said that. He had argued for transfer. Omar heard the transfer argument as a way of saying something else. His guess was right, and the conversation changed. Even if Omar had been wrong, the brother would have said "no, that's not it, what I am saying is..." and the meeting would still have shifted.

7.3 Reflections Of Feeling

In end of life care, the feelings in the room are often large and close to the surface. Grief, fear, anger, guilt, exhaustion, love, relief, dread. A skilled clinician learns to reflect these feelings directly, naming them rather than talking around them.

The basic structure of a feeling reflection is "you are feeling X because Y." You do not need to say the word "feeling." You can say "you are scared," "you are furious," "you are relieved," "you are heartbroken." Naming the feeling out loud does something important. It tells the person they are not alone with it. It also often gives them permission to feel it more fully, which paradoxically moves them through it faster.

Many clinicians avoid reflecting feelings because they are afraid of making things worse. This is almost always an illusion. The feeling is already in the room. Not naming it does not make it smaller, it just makes the person feel invisible with it. Naming a feeling does not cause it, any more than pointing out a thunderstorm causes the rain.

Reflections of feeling at end of life:

"You are terrified that this is really happening."

"You are furious at the doctors, and at the cancer, and at me, and I think at yourself too."

"You feel relieved, and you feel terrible for feeling relieved."

"This is the worst thing that has ever happened to you."

Notice that several of these reflections name feelings the person might be ashamed of. The daughter who feels relief when her mother finally dies is often ashamed of that relief. When a clinician names it as a normal part of caring for someone for a long time, the shame loosens. When nobody names it, the shame calcifies into something the daughter will carry for years.

One caution. Do not reflect feelings you do not believe are actually there. If a patient seems calm and you reflect "you must be so scared," you have imposed your expectation on their experience. They may be scared. They may not. Ask before you assume. "How are you feeling about this?" is often a better move than a reflection that guesses at an emotion you have not verified.

7.4 A Real Example

Meet Fatima. She was a hospice social worker in her fifth year. Her patient was a 71 year old man named Hassan with end stage COPD. His wife Yuki had been the primary caregiver for three years. On a Wednesday afternoon, Fatima met with Yuki while Hassan slept.

Yuki said, "The hospice nurse came yesterday and said he might not have much longer. A week maybe. I don't know what to do with that."

Fatima could have said "that must be so hard" (reassurance, not reflection). She could have said "you are dealing with a lot" (too simple, missed the weight). She could have started teaching about signs of imminent death (problem solving when none was asked for).

Instead she said, "You have been waiting for this for three years, and now that it might actually be here, you don't know how to be ready."

Yuki stared at her. Then she said, "Yes. That is it. I thought I was ready. I am not ready."

Fatima did not rush to fix this. She said, "Tell me what ready would have looked like."

Yuki talked for twenty minutes. About the things she had imagined saying. About the last trip they had meant to take. About the way she had been practicing for this for three years and still felt surprised. By the end, she was not fixed. She was not settled. But she was less alone with what she was feeling.

What this means for you: A complex reflection often works by naming the contradiction a person is living. Yuki had been preparing for Hassan's death and was still not ready. Both things were true. Fatima named both, and the naming itself gave Yuki a way to talk about it.

7.5 Double Sided Reflections

A **double sided reflection** captures both sides of a person's ambivalence at the same time. It is a specific type of complex reflection, and it is one of the most useful moves in palliative care because so many patients and families are of two minds about so many things.

The structure is: "You are X, and you are also Y." Both X and Y are things the person has said or implied. The reflection does not pick one side. It holds both.

Examples:

"You want him to keep fighting, and you also don't want him to suffer anymore."

"You know the chemo is not working, and you are not ready to stop."

"You want to take her home, and you are terrified of what will happen when you do."

"You want hospice, and you are afraid of what it means that you want it."

What double sided reflections do is prevent the patient from feeling they have to pick a side to please you. When you reflect only one side ("you know the chemo is not working"), you have amplified that side, which can push the patient toward a decision. When you reflect both sides, you have affirmed that they are allowed to feel both, which lets them think more clearly.

In MI with equipoise, double sided reflections are the core move. They are how you stay neutral while still actively engaging with what the person is saying. Miller and Rollnick recommend that when reflecting ambivalence, clinicians end with the side that seems to hold more change talk, because the order matters (Miller and Rollnick, 2023). "You are tired, and you want to keep going" ends on the persistence. "You want to keep going, and you are tired" ends on the exhaustion. If you are in non directive mode, alternate the ending across reflections so you do not steer. If you are in directive mode and the change you are supporting is medically clear, end on the side that supports it.

7.6 Another Real Example

Meet David. He was a palliative medicine nurse practitioner at a large academic hospital. His patient was Mrs. Antonescu, a 78 year old woman with advanced heart failure. She had been in and out of the hospital four times in six months. Her son Andrei had flown in from Chicago for this admission.

Andrei said in a family meeting: "I think we should try everything. She is tough. She has come back from worse. But I also see her suffering. I don't know what she would want."

A clinician in the righting reflex would have said something like, "It sounds like she is getting tired. Maybe it is time to focus on comfort." That is picking a side.

David said, "You love your mother and you want to give her every chance. You also see her hurting and you do not want her to keep going through this. Both of those things can be true at the same time."

Andrei was quiet for a long time. Then he said, "How do I know which one is right?"

David said, "Sometimes the answer is not one or the other. Sometimes it is trying to find what your mother would say if she could talk right now."

Andrei said, "She would say 'enough.' She has been telling me she has had enough for a year. I just did not want to hear her."

The family meeting shifted. They stopped trying to decide between fighting and comforting. They started asking what Mrs. Antonescu herself had said. The plan that emerged fit what she had been asking for all along.

What this means for you: Double sided reflections give people permission to feel what they are feeling without having to justify it. Once they do not have to defend a side, they can often hear what they already know. Andrei knew what his mother wanted. He needed someone to hold both of his feelings at once so he could stop fighting one of them.

7.7 Amplified Reflections

An **amplified reflection** takes what the person said and overstates it slightly, usually to allow the person to pull back. This is a specialized tool. Used well, it can crack open a stuck conversation. Used poorly, it fcels sarcastic or manipulative.

Example. A patient says, "I don't think I need hospice yet." An amplified reflection might be: "You are doing well enough right now that hospice would not add anything."

Notice what is happening. The clinician has taken the patient's statement and pushed it a little further. The patient now has to decide if they agree with the pushed version. If the pushed version goes too far (they are not actually "doing well enough"), the patient often pulls back and explains why they are in fact struggling. That is change talk, produced by the patient themselves.

Other examples:

Patient: "The morphine is too strong." Amplified reflection: "You are managing your pain just fine without it."

Family member: "Mom does not want to know her prognosis." Amplified reflection: "She would rather not have any information about what is coming."

These amplified reflections invite the listener to correct a slightly exaggerated version of what they said. When they correct, they often articulate a more nuanced version of their own position, which usually moves the conversation.

Amplified reflections require a particular tone. If you say it with any edge of sarcasm or challenge, it lands as mockery. The tone has to be genuinely curious, as if you are just checking that you have understood. Practice this out loud before you try it in a room with a family. The wrong tone can do real damage.

Amplified reflections are also not the first move. They work when you have already built rapport through simple and complex reflections and when the person trusts that you are on their side. Leading with an amplified reflection in a first visit will backfire. It is a tool for later in the conversation, after the relational ground is solid.

The rule of thumb: amplified reflections are powerful, occasional, and expensive if misused. Use them sparingly. When in doubt, go with a complex or double sided reflection instead.

7.8 When It Does Not Work

The most common failure with reflections is that they sound wooden. The clinician has read about reflections and is trying to produce them, but the words come out as a technique being performed rather than a response to what the person actually said. The family member hears it and knows they are being reflected at.

Three things to try when this happens:

1. Drop the word "sounds." Most wooden reflections start with "it sounds like..." That phrase telegraphs that you are using a technique. Just say what you heard. "You are tired." "You don't want him to suffer." "You are scared." Direct statements land cleaner than "sounds like" introductions. 2. When you reflect, say the thing you actually believe the person is feeling, not the thing you think is safest. A safe reflection of a scared patient might be "this is hard for you." A real reflection might be "you are terrified." The real one is scary to offer and almost always more effective. 3. If you catch yourself producing a reflection on autopilot, stop. Say, "I am trying to figure out what you are actually saying. Help me." That is more honest than a robotic reflection, and it usually gets a real answer.

A second failure mode is reflecting too much. If every single clinician response is a reflection, the conversation starts to feel strange, and the patient begins to notice that you never add anything. Reflections are the most common MI move, but they are not the only move. Mix them with open questions and occasional information sharing. A good ratio in MI work is roughly one reflection for each question, with complex reflections outnumbering simple ones at least slightly. If you are reflecting on every turn, take a breath and let the conversation breathe.

7.9 One More Look

Reflections are the most used and least flashy MI skill, and they are the single most powerful thing you can do in an end of life conversation. They do work that advice, reassurance, and information giving cannot do. Simple reflections confirm you heard. Complex reflections capture what is underneath the spoken words.

Feeling reflections name the emotion directly instead of talking around it.

Double sided reflections hold ambivalence without picking a side, which lets the patient or family think more clearly about what they actually want. Amplified reflections occasionally push a statement slightly further to invite a pullback, producing change talk from the patient themselves, but they require tone and timing and should be used sparingly.

Aim for one reflection for every question you ask. Aim for at least four of every ten reflections to be complex rather than simple. Practice naming feelings directly, including the hard ones. When your reflections feel wooden, drop "it sounds like" and just say the thing. When you reflect wrong, the correction you get is worth more than a right guess would have been.

The next chapter moves to the fourth of the OARS skills. **Summaries** are how you pull multiple strands of a conversation together, build coherence across visits, and help a family meeting find its way from chaos to clarity. You have seen Omar do one at the end of his meeting. The next chapter shows how.

Chapter 8: Summaries That Build Coherence

Isabella, a hospice nurse in her eleventh year, walked into a family meeting that was already off the rails. The patient was a 79 year old man named Miguel with advanced dementia, admitted to the skilled nursing facility six weeks ago. He had stopped eating three days earlier. His five adult children were fighting about a feeding tube.

The oldest son wanted the tube. The middle daughter did not. The youngest son was on FaceTime from Seattle and kept cutting out. The two middle kids were crying. The facility medical director had already left the meeting once to take a call. The social worker was frazzled. The chaplain had not been able to get a word in.

Isabella had been listening for twenty minutes. She finally said, "Can I try to say back what I have been hearing from each of you, just to see if I have it right?"

She took two minutes. She named what each person had said. She included the contradictions without resolving them. She ended with, "What everyone in this room seems to agree on is that you love him and you do not want him to suffer. You disagree about what that means for the feeding tube. Did I get anyone wrong?"

The room was quiet. The older son said, "That is exactly right."

The conversation that followed was different. Nobody was fighting to be heard anymore, because they had been heard. Within fifteen minutes, the family had agreed on a time limited trial of enteral feeding with clear criteria for stopping. Nobody walked out of the meeting feeling overridden.

Isabella's summary did not add any new information. It organized the information that was already in the room. That is what a good summary does, and it is the most underused tool in palliative care communication.

This chapter is about summaries: how to link them across visits, how to use them transitionally during goals of care conversations, how to deploy them in family meetings, how to write them so they invite next steps without pressure, and how to capture them in the medical record.

8.1 Linking Summaries Across Visits

A **linking summary** connects the current visit to prior ones. It tells the patient or family "I remember what we talked about last time, and I am bringing that into what we are doing now." This kind of summary is especially important in hospice and palliative care, where the patient may see three or four different team members across a week.

A good linking summary has three elements. It recalls what was said last time. It connects that content to something current. It invites the patient to update the picture.

Example: "When I was here Tuesday, you were telling me that your pain was better in the mornings but getting worse by dinner. You also said the nausea was making you skip lunch. How has that been since I saw you?"

This is not a fancy move. It is the kind of thing a thoughtful friend does when you catch up after a few days. In clinical settings, though, it is rare. Most clinicians start each visit fresh, as if they have never met the patient, because they are pressed for time and because they are relying on the chart to remind them of details that do not stick in their heads.

The reason linking summaries matter so much is that they signal continuity. The patient knows they are not a new story every time. For families who are telling the same story to a new nurse every few days, the experience of being remembered is therapeutic in itself.

A practical tip. Write one sentence at the end of each visit note that you will want to remember next time. Not a clinical detail. Something more specific. "Patient mentioned his daughter's graduation is in three weeks." "Wife is not sleeping because she checks his breathing every hour." "Son from Seattle arriving Friday, will want to be involved in decisions." On your next visit, read that sentence before you walk in. Bring it up. The whole interaction will change.

8.2 Transitional Summaries

A **transitional summary** pulls together a stretch of conversation and uses the summary itself as a bridge to the next part. It is especially useful in goals of care conversations, where you have been exploring values and now need to move toward a plan.

The structure is: "Let me see if I have understood you. You have told me X, Y, and Z. Given what you have said, it makes sense to think about..."

Example: "Let me take a moment. You have told me that being home with your husband matters more to you than anything else. You have told me the hospital trips have been hard on both of you. You have told me the IV nutrition is not giving you much quality of life but you have been scared to stop it. Given those things, it makes sense to ask how we can build a plan that keeps you home and reduces the trips, and to look at the IV nutrition together. Is that the conversation you want to have next?"

Notice what this does. It compresses a fifteen minute conversation into twenty seconds of organized reflection. It tells the patient you have been tracking. It proposes a direction, but it frames the direction as emerging from what the patient said, not from what the clinician wanted. And it ends with a question that lets the patient correct or redirect.

Transitional summaries are how you move a conversation forward without imposing. Without them, goals of care conversations often meander for an hour and end without a clear next step. With them, the conversation feels purposeful without feeling pushed.

The Serious Illness Conversation Guide from Ariadne Labs includes a recommendation to use this kind of summary before making a recommendation (Bernacki and Block, 2014). You synthesize what the patient has said, then you offer a recommendation framed as "given what you told me, I wonder if X would fit." This structure consistently tests as more acceptable to patients than recommendations delivered without the preceding summary (Paladino et al., 2019).

8.3 Family Meeting Summaries

In a family meeting, a **collecting summary** is the move Isabella used in the opening. You pull together what multiple people have said and reflect it back to the room. This is one of the most useful single skills in family meeting facilitation.

A collecting summary has to do several things. It has to name each major speaker's position fairly. It has to hold contradictions without papering over them. It has to find what is shared, if anything. And it has to invite correction.

Example structure: "Let me try to say back what I have been hearing. [Name], you are saying X because Y matters to you. [Name], you are saying A because B matters to you. What I am hearing both of you agree on is that you love him and you want what is best. You disagree about what that looks like. Did I get anyone wrong?"

Three things make this work. First, you use names. People feel heard differently when their name is said. Second, you connect the position to the underlying value. Saying "you want the feeding tube" is a position. Saying "you want the feeding tube because you want to know you tried everything" is a reason, and reasons build understanding in a way positions do not. Third, you end with an invitation to correct. If you got it wrong, the room will tell you, and the correction is almost always useful.

The magic of a collecting summary is that once people feel heard, they stop fighting to be heard. Most family meeting conflict is not really about the medical decision. It is about people fearing that their perspective will be overridden. When a skilled facilitator names each perspective accurately, the room relaxes. Once it relaxes, people can actually think about the decision.

One risk to avoid. A collecting summary should not try to resolve the disagreement. It names the positions and the underlying values, and stops there. If you use the summary to argue for one side ("so given that you all want what is best, it really does sound like the feeding tube makes sense"), you have used the technique as a weapon, and the family will feel it. Stop at the naming. The resolution comes later, from the family itself, once they are no longer arguing to be seen.

8.4 A Real Example

Meet Raj. He was a palliative medicine physician in his eighth year. His patient was a 64 year old woman named Amara with metastatic breast cancer. Her first goals of care conversation had lasted thirty five minutes and had surfaced a great deal. Near the end, Raj did this summary:

"Let me see if I have you right. You have told me that the chemotherapy has been harder than anything you have been through. You have told me that you were initially willing to try anything because you wanted to be there for your daughter's wedding in June. You have told me that even if you make the wedding, you are not sure you want to keep going after that. And you have told me that you have not talked to your daughter about any of this because you do not want to worry her before the wedding. Is that right?"

Amara said, "Yes. That is exactly where I am."

Raj said, "Given all of that, there are two conversations we could have next. One is about how to get you through to June with as much quality as possible. The other is about how to start the conversation with your daughter. Which one do you want to do first?"

Amara said, "The one with my daughter. I have been trying to figure out how to say this for months."

Raj spent the next twenty five minutes not on medical planning but on helping Amara plan what to say to her daughter, when to say it, and who might help her. The summary made that possible. Without the summary, the conversation would have drifted toward the medical details. With the summary, Amara got to pick where to go next. She picked what she actually needed.

What this means for you: A summary at the end of a rich conversation gives the patient a chance to direct what happens next. You do the organizing work. They do the choosing. That division of labor is what makes the conversation feel collaborative rather than doctor led.

8.5 Summaries That Invite Without Pushing

A good summary ends with an invitation, not a conclusion. The clinician has synthesized. The patient now gets to say what the synthesis means. The invitation is how you keep the summary from becoming a verdict.

Compare these two endings to the same summary.

Ending one: "So it is pretty clear that we should transition to comfort focused care."

Ending two: "Given what you have told me, what feels like the right next step for you?"

Ending one concluded. It closed the conversation. The patient either agrees or has to push back against the clinician's conclusion. Ending two synthesized without concluding. It kept the choosing inside the patient's own frame.

The specific invitational endings that tend to work:

"What feels right to you?"

"What should we do with all of that?"

"Where do you want to go from here?"

"What would be most helpful to talk about next?"

"Is there anything I am missing?"

You will notice these are open questions. A good summary bridges to an open question. The pattern is: reflection, reflection, reflection, summary, open question. That rhythm keeps the conversation in the patient's direction while giving them the organizing help they need.

One more move. Sometimes the most honest ending to a summary is "I notice I do not know what you want to do with this, and I do not want to guess. What are you thinking?" This is useful when you are being pulled toward a particular recommendation and you are not sure you should be. Naming your own uncertainty is often more respectful than pretending to be sure.

8.6 Writing The Summary Into The Chart

Everything you have learned in this chapter also applies to documentation. A good chart note is a kind of summary: of what the patient said, what values emerged, what decisions were made, and what remains open. Most clinical notes fail at this because they are written in medical shorthand that strips the humanity out of the conversation.

The practical move is to include, in your note, one or two direct quotes from the patient in their own words. Not a clinical translation. Their actual words. "Patient states, 'I want to be home for my granddaughter's birthday in May.'" This kind of quote does two things. It preserves the patient's voice in the record so that other team members encounter it as the patient said it. And it makes the note a reference document for future goals of care work, because the quote itself is what everyone will come back to.

Another move is to include a short values section separate from the medical assessment. Something like:

Patient's stated priorities: being home, not returning to the hospital, being there for the May birthday. Patient's stated concerns: pain, being a burden on daughter, running out of time to talk to her sister. Patient's decision today: continue home hospice, no hospitalization for acute symptoms, decision about sister left open for now.

This format makes the note useful to every clinician who reads it. It also protects the patient's wishes against the drift that tends to happen when different team members each make their own interpretation of what the patient wanted.

A final note on documentation. If your system uses the Serious Illness Conversation Guide or a similar structured tool, the guide provides a documentation template that mirrors the conversation structure. Using that template consistently builds organizational memory across clinicians and shifts. If your system does not use a formal template, you can build your own using the categories above: priorities, concerns, decisions made, decisions open.

8.7 Another Real Example

Meet Nicole. She was a palliative care clinical nurse specialist at a children's hospital. Her patient was a 14 year old boy named Diego with a relapsed brain tumor. His parents and his oncologist had been in a conflict for two weeks. The oncologist wanted to offer a phase one trial. The parents were leaning against it. Diego himself had not been included in the conversations.

Nicole convened a meeting. After forty five minutes of careful listening, she said:

"Let me try to put this together. Dr. [oncologist], you are saying the phase one trial is a legitimate option because it has produced some responses in similar tumors, and you want Diego and the family to have the choice. Mr. and Mrs. [parents], you are saying that Diego has been through three years of treatment and you do not want him to spend his last months in a research protocol if the chance of benefit is small. All of you seem to agree that the final call should take Diego's own preferences into account. What I am not hearing is what Diego has said about this. Have we asked him?"

The oncologist and the parents looked at each other. The mother said, "We have not. We have been trying to decide for him."

Nicole said, "Would you want me to talk with him?"

They agreed. Nicole met with Diego alone that afternoon. He said he did not want the trial. He wanted to go home. He wanted to play his video games with his brother. He wanted to see his grandmother one more time. He had been waiting for someone to ask him.

What this means for you: Sometimes a summary reveals what is missing rather than what is present. Nicole's summary did not resolve the conflict between oncologist and parents. It named what neither of them had done: ask the patient. Summaries can be diagnostic as well as integrative. When you summarize what you have heard, you often see what has not been said.

8.8 When It Does Not Work

The most common way summaries fail is that the clinician uses the summary to settle something that should not yet be settled. You have listened to a patient's complicated feelings about stopping chemo, and at the end you say, "So it sounds like you are ready to stop." The patient may not be ready. You have put words in their mouth. If they were not ready, they now have to push back against you instead of against their own ambivalence. You have made it harder, not easier.

Three things to try:

1. Before you summarize, ask yourself: am I summarizing to help the patient think, or am I summarizing to move them toward a decision I want? If the latter, stop. Ask an open question instead. 2. When you summarize, include contradictions. If the patient has said two things that do not match, your summary should include both. Picking the side you prefer is not a summary, it is a vote. 3. End with an invitation, not a conclusion. "What do you want to do with all of that?" is an invitation. "So I think we should move forward with hospice" is a conclusion. The first keeps the choosing with the patient. The second takes it.

A second common failure is the summary that is too long. If your summary takes three minutes to deliver, nobody in the room is going to track it. A good summary is compressed. Hit the essentials. Leave the rest for later.

A third failure is summarizing without having actually listened. If the clinician's summary does not ring true, the patient will feel dismissed, and the remaining conversation will suffer. You cannot summarize what you have not tracked. The only fix for this is listening more closely earlier in the conversation, so the summary has something real to organize.

8.9 The Main Ideas

Summaries are the organizing work of a conversation. Linking summaries connect the current visit to prior ones and signal that the patient is remembered. Transitional summaries compress a stretch of conversation and bridge to what comes next. Collecting summaries in family meetings pull together multiple perspectives and hold contradictions without resolving them prematurely.

Good summaries use names, connect positions to underlying values, and end with an invitation rather than a conclusion. They put the choosing in the patient's hands after you have done the organizing work. They also translate into documentation, where direct patient quotes and explicit values sections preserve the patient's voice in the record.

The most important discipline with summaries is avoiding the temptation to use them as verdicts. A summary should open the conversation, not close it. When you feel yourself reaching for a summary to settle something, pause, and consider if a question would be more honest.

The fifth and final chapter of Part II goes deeper into one specific application of all four OARS skills. It is about eliciting what matters most to a patient: the values work that is the heart of goals of care conversations. You will meet the techniques that turn "what do you want" from a useless question into a productive one.

Chapter 9: Eliciting What Matters Most

Mr. Castellanos was 84 years old, a widower, a retired machinist who had spent his whole adult life in the same small house in Lowell, Massachusetts. He had been diagnosed with heart failure six years ago. He had been hospitalized three times in the last eight months. His cardiologist had asked him, at every visit for two years, if he wanted to talk about advance directives. Every time, Mr. Castellanos had said no.

His granddaughter Isabella had brought him to a new primary care appointment. The nurse practitioner, a woman named Amara, had been briefed by the cardiology office. They warned her he would not discuss it. She had tried twice herself in previous visits.

On the third visit, Amara did something different. She put the advance directive packet away. She sat down next to Mr. Castellanos. She said, "Mr. Castellanos, when you wake up on a good day, what do you do first?"

He looked at her. He said, "I make coffee. Then I go out on the porch and look at the birds in the feeder. My wife put the feeder up thirty years ago."

Amara said, "Tell me about the birds."

He talked for about five minutes. About the cardinals that came in pairs. About the hawk that had shown up last fall. About his wife putting the feeder up the first spring after they moved in.

Then Amara said, "If your heart started to fail again, and the doctors wanted to send you to the ICU to try to save you, what would you want to happen?"

Mr. Castellanos said, without hesitating, "I want to die on my porch. I want Isabella to hold my hand. I do not want to die in a room full of machines. I do not want anyone breaking my ribs to bring me back."

Amara wrote it down. She read it back. He signed the form.

The whole conversation took twenty eight minutes. The cardiologist had tried for two years. The difference was not what Amara asked about the heart. It was what she asked about the birds.

This chapter is about **eliciting values**, which is the core work of goals of care and advance care planning. You will learn why values have to come before preferences, and preferences before decisions. You will meet the "best day and hardest day" method. You will see how life review functions as a clinical tool. You will learn to use the Serious Illness Conversation Guide through an MI lens. And you will learn what to do with what you elicit, because gathering values is only useful if you do something with them.

9.1 Values Before Preferences

Most advance care planning conversations fail because they start in the wrong place. The clinician opens with preferences. "Do you want to be resuscitated?" "Do you want a feeding tube?" "Do you want to be intubated?" The patient has no context for answering these questions. They pick something to make the conversation end. The form gets signed. The form does not reflect what the patient actually wants.

A better sequence is values first, then preferences, then decisions.

Values are the underlying things that matter to a person. Being at home. Being pain free. Being mentally present for important events. Not being a burden. Seeing particular people. Doing particular things.

Preferences are the specific care choices that flow from those values. Because I want to be at home, I prefer hospice. Because I want to be mentally present, I prefer less sedating pain management.

Because I do not want to be resuscitated into a worse state, I prefer DNR.

Decisions are the concrete agreements that go into the record and drive care. Enroll in hospice. Document the DNR. Arrange home care.

If you start with decisions, the patient often makes the wrong one because they do not yet know what they are choosing. If you start with preferences, they often pick options that sound reasonable but that do not match their actual values. If you start with values, the rest follows more naturally because you are now building on what actually matters to them.

This is why Mr. Castellanos answered the ICU question in thirty seconds after two years of silence. Once he was connected to what he valued (the porch, the birds, his wife's feeder, Isabella's hand), the question about the ICU had a context. Without that context, the question was abstract and unanswerable. With the context, the answer was obvious.

The clinical move is simple and requires discipline. Do not ask about care choices until you have spent time asking about the person's life. This feels inefficient. It is actually faster.

9.2 The Best Day And Hardest Day Elicitation

One of the most useful tools in values elicitation is a pair of questions: "What does a good day look like for you now?" and "What does a hard day look like?"

These questions work because they are concrete. Abstract values questions ("what is important to you") sometimes get abstract answers. The best day and hardest day questions get detail, because the person has to think in specifics to answer.

Examples of what patients actually say:

"A good day is when I can walk to the mailbox without getting short of breath. A hard day is when I can't get out of bed and my daughter has to help me use the bathroom."

"A good day is when I am not nauseated. I can sit in the living room and read. A hard day is when the nausea starts in the morning and nothing helps and I spend the day staring at the ceiling."

"A good day is when my husband and I can watch our show together. A hard day is when he comes to visit and I am too out of it to know he is there."

Notice what these answers tell you. They tell you what the patient can still do on their best days. They tell you what they cannot do on their worst days. They tell you what is worth fighting for (good days with enough of them) and what is worth preventing (hard days that become the norm). They are the raw material of a goals of care plan.

Once you have this, you can ask follow up questions that are specific and actionable. "When the hard days outnumber the good days, what do you want us to do?" "What would count as enough good days to be worth it?" "If treatment took away your ability to have any good days, would you want to continue?" These questions are answerable because the patient now has a picture of good and hard days in their head.

The best day and hardest day elicitation takes about ten minutes. It surfaces more useful values information than any checklist. It works for patients who have never thought about advance care planning and for patients who have been thinking about it for years.

9.3 Life Review

Life review is a specific technique that invites a patient to tell the story of their life. It sounds strange in a clinical context. It is one of the most powerful values elicitation tools that exists, and it produces clinical information that no other method produces.

The basic prompt is simple. "I would like to know a little about your life, not just your illness. Tell me about yourself."

Some patients will start with their childhood. Some will start with their career. Some will start with their family. It does not matter where they start. Let them talk. Ask follow up questions that show you are listening. Do not redirect to medical topics.

What comes out in life review tells you what the patient has been oriented around their whole life. A woman who spends twenty minutes talking about her career as a teacher is telling you that contribution and meaning through work matter. A man who spends twenty minutes talking about his children is telling you that family is central. A veteran who tells war stories is often telling you something about honor, duty, or survival that shapes how he will face death.

This information becomes directly relevant to clinical decisions. The teacher who has oriented her life around contribution often wants the last weeks to have some form of contribution in them: leaving letters, recording stories, teaching someone. The family man often wants presence and time with people more than treatment. The veteran often has a specific relationship to pain and suffering that affects how he wants to be medicated.

Life review does two other things at once. It builds a relationship of trust with the clinician faster than almost any other intervention. And it is often therapeutic in itself. Many older patients have not been asked about their lives in years. The experience of being asked, and of being listened to, is often the first thing that reduces their distress in the clinical setting.

If you are thinking "I do not have time for this in a twenty minute visit," you are right. Life review does not fit into a twenty minute visit. It does fit into a first home hospice admission visit, or a chaplain visit, or a social work visit, or a deliberately scheduled conversation. It does not have to be long. Ten minutes of real life review produces more clinical value than thirty minutes of standard history taking.

9.4 A Real Example

Meet Marcus. He was a palliative care social worker in his fourth year. His new patient was Mrs. Okafor, a 79 year old Nigerian woman with metastatic colon cancer. Her chart described her as "non engaged with advance care planning." She had refused to sign any forms. The oncologist had asked Marcus to "try to get her on board."

Marcus did not mention forms. He sat with her for forty minutes. He asked her about her life. She told him about coming to the United States from Nigeria in 1971, about raising four children while working as a nurse's aide, about the church she had attended for thirty nine years, about the grandchildren she had. She showed him pictures.

At minute thirty two, Marcus asked her, "If you could choose how your last weeks go, what would they look like?"

Mrs. Okafor said, "I want to die in my house. I want my pastor to come and pray with me. I want my children to be there. I do not want to go back to the hospital. The hospital is a cold place to die."

Marcus said, "Is there anything you want us to make sure does not happen?"

She said, "I do not want to be cut open again. I do not want tubes. If I am dying, I want to die with my body as it is."

Marcus wrote it down. He read it back to her. He asked if she wanted the care plan to reflect what she had just said. She said yes.

He filled in the advance directive form using her words. She signed it.

What this means for you: A patient who has refused to "do" advance care planning for two years is not refusing to have values about her own care. She is refusing a format that does not feel like hers. When you get the format out of the way and ask about her life first, the care planning often happens naturally, because the values were already there waiting to be asked about.

9.5 The SICG Through An MI Lens

The Serious Illness Conversation Guide developed by Ariadne Labs is the most widely used structured tool for goals of care conversations. It has been implemented by more than three hundred organizations and used in the training of over thirteen thousand clinicians (Ariadne Labs, 2023). The guide has strong evidence behind it: a cluster randomized trial in outpatient oncology found that patients whose clinicians used it reported lower rates of anxiety and depression (Bernacki et al., 2019).

The guide has six sections: set up the conversation, assess illness understanding and information preferences, share prognosis according to preferences, explore patient values and goals, make a recommendation, and close the conversation. In practice, the core of the guide is a series of questions, including:

"What is your understanding of where you are with your illness?" "How much information about what is likely to be ahead would you like from me?" "If your health situation worsens, what are your most important goals?" "What are your biggest fears and worries about the future with your health?" "What gives you strength as you think about the future with your illness?" "What abilities are so critical to your life that you cannot imagine living without them?" "If you become sicker, how much are you willing to go through for the possibility of gaining more time?" "How much does your family know about your priorities and wishes?"

Using the guide through an MI lens means integrating these questions with the OARS skills you have learned. After a patient answers the understanding question, you reflect what you heard before moving to the next question. After they name fears, you do not rush past them; you reflect, maybe ask a complex reflection, sit with the feeling before proceeding. Before making a recommendation, you summarize what they have said, connect the recommendation to their stated values, and offer it with an invitation to push back.

The guide is not a checklist. If you treat it as a checklist, you will race through the questions, collect answers, and miss the actual conversation. If you treat it as a structure that holds a real MI conversation, the guide and MI amplify each other.

One specific move. When a patient gives a rich answer to one of the guide's questions, do not immediately move to the next question. Reflect. Ask a follow up. Let the conversation expand around the rich answer. The guide is there to make sure you hit the major domains, not to control the pace. A great goals of care conversation using the guide rarely goes through the questions in order. It moves fluidly, returns to earlier topics, and gets deeper on the questions that matter most to this particular patient.

9.6 Another Real Example

Meet David. He was a hospice medical director who had been using the SICG for six years. His patient was Mr. Blackwell, a 68 year old man with advanced prostate cancer. David had forty five minutes scheduled.

David started with the first SICG question: "What is your understanding of where you are with your illness?"

Mr. Blackwell said, "I know I'm dying. Doc says I might have a few months. But I'm trying not to think about it too much."

David reflected: "You know what's coming, and you are trying to keep it at arm's length."

Mr. Blackwell nodded.

David asked: "What are you most afraid of about the future with your health?"

Mr. Blackwell said, "Pain. I don't want to die in pain. I saw my dad die that way."

David did not move to the next question. He said, "Your dad's pain is still with you."

Mr. Blackwell's eyes filled up. He talked for fifteen minutes about his father, who had died of colon cancer in 1987. He talked about watching his mother hold his father's hand while he moaned. He talked about promising himself he would never die that way.

David said, "So when we talk about how your last weeks go, the top priority is making sure your pain is controlled. Is there anything else as important as that to you?"

Mr. Blackwell said, "I want to be home. I want my dogs with me."

David said, "Pain controlled, at home, with your dogs. Those are the three things."

Mr. Blackwell said, "Yes. Those are the three things."

David wrote them into the plan of care. He called the hospice nurses and the home aide team. The pain management plan was built around those three priorities. Mr. Blackwell died four months later, at home, with his dogs, and without pain. His daughter wrote David a letter afterward saying that her father had had the death her grandfather did not.

What this means for you: The SICG gave the structure. MI gave the depth. When David heard the reference to Mr. Blackwell's father, he did not move on. He reflected and asked, and the conversation opened into the story that was driving everything. The plan that came from that conversation was specifically tailored because it was built on what the patient had actually said. Generic goals of care plans deliver generic care. Values specific plans deliver values specific care.

9.7 What To Do With What You Elicit

Eliciting values is useless if the values do not change anything. Once you have them, three things need to happen.

First, document them clearly. Use the patient's own words when possible. Include a values section in your note that lists priorities, concerns, and decisions made. Use direct quotes. Make sure the note is readable by any clinician who might see the patient next.

Second, translate the values into the care plan. If the patient has said pain control is the top priority, the pain management plan should reflect that. If they have said being home matters most, the plan should avoid hospitalization for anything that can be managed at home. If they have said they want their dogs with them, make sure the facility accommodates that. The translation from values to plan is your responsibility. It does not happen on its own.

Third, communicate the values to the rest of the team. In interdisciplinary team meetings, share not just the medical status but the values. "Mr. Blackwell's three priorities are pain control, being home, and his dogs. Please keep those in mind when you are making decisions about his care." The hospice aide who is bathing him needs to know the dogs matter. The nurse who is making pain management calls needs to know pain is the number one concern. The social worker who is planning family meetings needs to know being home is non negotiable.

When the values actually shape the care, the patient experiences something rare in the medical system: they experience being known. Their care does not feel like a protocol being applied to them. It feels like a plan that was built for them specifically, because it was.

This is the point of all the skills in Part II. Open questions, affirmations, reflections, summaries, and values elicitation are not ends in themselves. They are tools for building care that fits the person in front of you. The next five chapters, in Part III, take you into the specific hard conversations where you will use these skills most intensively: introducing hospice, breaking bad news, discussing prognosis, establishing goals of care, and talking about feared medicines.

9.8 When It Does Not Work

The most common failure mode in values elicitation is that the clinician asks a values question, gets a rich answer, and then moves on without doing anything with it. The patient said something that mattered. The clinician said "thank you for sharing that" and shifted back to medical topics. The values answer died on the floor.

Three things to try:

1. When a patient gives you a values answer, reflect it before you do anything else. "Being home with your dogs matters more to you than the treatment." The reflection tells the patient you heard. It also keeps the value present in the conversation rather than letting it slip away. 2. Write the patient's values in their own words in your note. Not "patient prefers home based care," but "patient states he wants to be home with his dogs when he dies." The patient's words have power that translated summaries do not. 3. Before you leave the visit, tell the patient what you are going to do with what they told you. "I am going to make sure the pain management team knows that pain control is your number one priority. I am going to

talk to the hospice nurses about making sure your dogs can stay with you." This closes the loop. The patient knows their answer landed.

A second failure is pushing for values answers when the patient is not ready. Some patients, on a particular day, cannot do values work. They are too symptomatic, too grieving, too overwhelmed. If you push, they will shut down. If that happens, do not interpret it as refusal of advance care planning. Come back another day. Say, "We can talk about this another time. Let me know when you are ready." Most patients will be ready eventually. Forcing the conversation on the wrong day often makes the right day harder to reach.

9.9 Where You Are Now

You have finished Part II. You have met the four OARS skills and their application to values elicitation. You know how to ask open questions that open hearts, how to give affirmations that do not ring hollow, how to offer reflections that do the work, and how to build summaries that organize what has been said without imposing what has not.

You know that values come before preferences and preferences before decisions. You have met the best day and hardest day elicitation, which surfaces specific and actionable information in about ten minutes. You have learned that life review is a clinical tool, not a social nicety. You have seen how the Serious Illness Conversation Guide works when used through an MI lens.

Most important, you know that eliciting values is only the beginning. Values have to become documentation. Documentation has to become care plans. Care plans have to become shared understanding across the team. When that full sequence happens, the patient experiences something almost every patient reports wanting: care that fits who they actually are.

Part III begins with the hardest conversations, starting with how to introduce hospice without triggering the feeling that everyone has given up. All the skills from Part II will be with you. You will use them in situations you have been dreading. You will find that they make those situations more bearable for everyone in the room, including you.

PART III: THE TOUGHEST CONVERSATIONS

Chapter 10: Introducing Hospice Without Losing Hope

Dr. Joseph Turner had been a family physician in rural Indiana for twenty one years. He knew his patients in a way that is rare in modern medicine. He had delivered their babies. He had treated their parents. He sat on the same church council as half of them. This is a story about one of his patients, and it is a story he told at a hospice continuing education event ten years after it happened.

The patient was a 57 year old farmer named Mr. Klein. Six months earlier, Mr. Klein had been diagnosed with metastatic esophageal cancer. His oncologist had tried two lines of chemotherapy. The tumor had grown through both. By the time Mr. Klein came to see Dr. Turner on a Tuesday in October, he was 40 pounds lighter, he was eating soft foods and still losing weight, and he could not walk from the parking lot to the exam room without resting.

Dr. Turner said, "Frank, I want to talk to you about hospice."

Mr. Klein said, "No."

Dr. Turner explained what hospice was. Mr. Klein said no again.

Dr. Turner explained that hospice did not mean giving up. Mr. Klein said no.

Dr. Turner talked about what his wife was going through. Mr. Klein said, "I'm not dying yet."

Dr. Turner tried every tool he had. He was honest. He was clear. He was kind. He offered specific benefits. He warned about specific harms. Over eight weeks and four visits, he tried to get Mr. Klein to say yes to hospice. Mr. Klein never did. Eventually he died in the ICU two days after a fall at home. His wife never forgave Dr. Turner for not "trying harder."

When Dr. Turner told this story at the education event, he said something that stuck with everyone in the room. He said, "I spent all my energy trying to convince him. I never once asked him what hospice meant to him. If I had, I think we might have gotten somewhere."

This chapter is about what Dr. Turner wishes he had known. You will learn why the word hospice triggers a defense reaction, how to prepare the ground before you mention the word, how to reframe hospice from cliff to layer, how to roll with resistance when it is genuinely a wall, and how the second and third conversations often matter more than the first.

10.1 Why Hospice Triggers Defense

The word "hospice" has associations that are not primarily clinical. For most patients and families, it means "my doctor has given up." It means "I am dying soon." It means "my people will watch me die." These associations have nothing to do with the actual Medicare hospice benefit, which is a set of services that can include skilled nursing, symptom management, counseling, chaplaincy, volunteer companionship, and respite care. But the associations came first, and the clinical reality comes second.

When you walk into a room and say "I want to talk to you about hospice," you have just activated the emotional file the patient has in their head. If their file is mostly dread and loss, they will react to the dread and loss, not to the services you are about to describe. You can talk for twenty minutes about the benefits of hospice. The patient is still living inside "my doctor has given up."

This is not irrationality. It is ordinary human cognition. We react to what words mean to us before we process what they mean technically. A patient who has watched a parent die in hospice thirty years ago, when hospice looked very different from today, has a specific memory shaping their reaction. A patient whose only association with hospice is a television drama has that reaction. A patient whose uncle was admitted to hospice two days before his death has an association with "last thing they do before you die" that is nearly unshakeable.

The research is consistent. Patients often equate hospice with giving up, and clinicians who introduce it in ways that reinforce this equivalence produce predictable refusals (Vig et al., 2010). Part of what is happening is that hospice is often introduced too late. A patient who first hears the word from their oncologist after three lines of failed chemotherapy will hear it as the thing that comes after the oncologist has run out of options. That timing teaches a meaning, and the meaning sticks.

Your job, before you use the word, is to understand what the word already means to this patient. You can do this with one question: "What do you know about hospice?" The answer will tell you which file you are activating. You can then work with that file before you add anything new.

10.2 Preparing The Soil

Before you plant the word, you prepare the soil. This means you do three things before the word hospice enters the conversation.

First, you elicit values. You have read Chapter 9.0. You know how to do this. You ask what matters to the patient, what a good day looks like, what they fear about the future. You listen. You reflect. By the time you consider mentioning hospice, you know something about this specific person.

Second, you establish a shared picture of the illness. Before anyone discusses hospice, patient and clinician need to be in roughly the same place about what the disease is doing. If you think they are dying and they think they are on the mend, any conversation about hospice will feel like a non sequitur. You ask what they understand. You correct gently, if correction is invited. You do not bludgeon them with prognostic facts. You help them arrive at a realistic picture in their own time.

Third, you ask what they know about hospice. This is the critical move that Dr. Turner missed. If you skip it, you will end up arguing against associations you do not even know the patient has. If you make it, you can address the specific fears, myths, and memories that are driving the reaction.

Here is what this can sound like in sequence.

"Tell me what matters most to you right now."

Pause. Listen. Reflect.

"What is your sense of where things are going with the illness?"

Pause. Listen. Reflect. Possibly share a little, with permission.

"What do you know about hospice?"

Pause. Listen. Reflect.

Only after this do you say anything of your own about hospice. By this point you are not introducing a new topic. You are connecting the patient's own values and understanding to a set of services that might fit. The conversation is already in their frame. You are not selling. You are joining.

This preparation takes time. It takes a visit. Sometimes it takes two or three visits. This is why the second and third conversations matter so much, which section 10.5 will return to.

10.3 Hospice As A Layer

The most useful reframe in this work is from "cliff" to "layer." A cliff is what the word hospice sounds like. A layer is what hospice actually is.

A cliff is a discrete event. You fall off it. You go from one thing (trying to beat the disease) to another thing (waiting to die). A layer is something added to what the patient already has. They are still their person, with their life, their relationships, their goals. Hospice is a set of additional resources that comes alongside them.

Concretely, hospice on top of their existing life adds a nurse who visits regularly, a social worker who helps with the hard conversations, a chaplain who can be present for spiritual questions, a home health aide who helps with bathing, and a twenty four hour phone line for symptom problems that come up at 3 a.m. None of those things replace anything the patient already has. They add to it.

The language you use matters. Compare these two statements.

"It is time to transition to hospice." "What if we added a layer of support on top of what you already have?"

The first assumes an ending. The second suggests an addition. Most patients respond differently to an addition than to an ending, even when the clinical situation is the same.

Other framings that tend to work:

"Hospice is not about stopping care. It is about changing who provides which parts of your care."

"You can think of hospice as a team that specializes in helping people be as comfortable as possible at home."

"Many people who sign up for hospice live longer than they expected, because they stop making the trips that were wearing them out."

This last one is not a sales line. It is supported by research. A study of Medicare patients with advanced cancer, heart failure, and COPD found that hospice enrollment was associated with slightly longer survival in several disease categories compared to matched controls, likely because of better symptom management and fewer hospital acquired problems (Connor et al., 2007). This does not mean hospice extends life in every case. It does mean the mental model of "hospice shortens your life" is not supported by the evidence.

Use any of these framings with discretion. If the patient's reaction to the word hospice is strong, lead with listening, not with a correction of their framing. Correcting a scared patient feels like argument, and argument increases the sustain talk that section 10.4 addresses.

10.4 Rolling With Resistance

You have prepared the soil. You have offered a layer framing. The patient still says no.

Now what.

Most clinicians, at this point, either give up or push harder. Both fail. The MI move is to roll with the resistance. You reflect what the patient is saying. You do not argue. You explore what is underneath the no.

"You are telling me you are not ready for that. Help me understand what that feels like from where you are sitting."

"That is a no, and I can hear how strong the no is. What is the strongest part of the no?"

"You do not want this. I am not going to talk you into it. I do want to understand, if you are willing to tell me, what you are most afraid of about hospice."

Each of these moves takes the pressure off the patient to defend their position. When the pressure is off, patients often explain their no in ways that surface the fear underneath. The fear is usually what you can actually address. The no is often a symptom of the fear, not the real thing.

Common fears under no:

"They will sedate me and I will lose time with my family."

"I will lose my doctor."

"My insurance will stop covering things."

"Signing means I have admitted I am dying."

"I will disappoint my children, who want me to keep fighting."

Each of these is a different conversation. The fear about sedation calls for a discussion of how symptom management actually works in hospice. The fear about losing the doctor calls for a clarification of how hospice teams coordinate with existing physicians. The fear about insurance calls for concrete information about the Medicare hospice benefit. The fear about disappointing children calls for something much harder, which is help planning a conversation with the children.

You cannot have any of these conversations until you know which fear you are in. Rolling with resistance is how you find out.

One more thing. When the patient says no, do not assume the no is about hospice. Sometimes the no is about everything. The patient is refusing to accept the whole situation, and saying no to hospice is one manifestation of refusing everything. In those cases, the hospice conversation has to wait. What the patient actually needs is help grieving the fact that they are dying. Hospice will come later, after the grief has moved.

10.5 The Second And Third Conversations

The research on hospice enrollment suggests that many patients who eventually enroll say no the first time it is offered (Casarett et al., 2005). The no is not final. It is the beginning of a process. The clinician who accepts the first no gracefully and leaves the door open often gets a yes on the second or third conversation.

What does gracefully mean. It means you do not pressure. You do not imply the patient is making a mistake. You do not hint at what will happen if they keep refusing. You acknowledge the no, thank them for being honest, and tell them you will be back.

"Okay. You are not ready for this today. I hear you. I am going to keep coming to see you, and we can talk about this again whenever you want to."

That sentence, delivered with real acceptance, is a bridge. The patient does not feel they have to defend against future pressure. They can actually think about what you said, because they are not busy resisting you.

The second conversation often happens when something has changed. A new symptom. A new decline. A family member who said something. The first conversation planted a seed. The second conversation finds the seed has sprouted.

When you return, do not start with hospice. Start with how they are doing. Ask what has changed. Listen. Often they will bring up the hospice question themselves. If they do not, and you sense an opening, you can gently revisit: "Last time we talked I mentioned hospice and you told me you were not ready. I am wondering if anything has shifted since then, or if you would like to ask any more questions about what it would look like."

Note what this does. It does not press for a decision. It opens a door. The patient can walk through or not, on their terms.

Some patients never say yes. They die without hospice. That is not necessarily a failure of your communication. It is sometimes a reflection of what that specific person needed to do with their dying, which may include not signing the form. Your job is to make the door available. What the patient walks through is theirs.

10.6 A Real Example

Meet Elena. She was a palliative care nurse practitioner in her seventh year, working in a community hospital in Baltimore. Her patient was Mr. Afolabi, a 72 year old retired school principal with metastatic prostate cancer. He had been offered hospice three times by his oncologist. He had said no each time.

Elena met him during an admission for uncontrolled pain. She did not mention hospice in their first conversation. She asked him about himself. He told her about thirty eight years of teaching. About his four children. About his wife, who had died nine years ago. About how he had been a strong man his whole life and did not know how to be anything else.

Elena said, "So being strong has been a big part of who you are."

He said, "Yes."

Elena said, "What do you know about hospice?"

He said, "It is what they call it when the doctors are done with you."

Elena said, "Tell me more about that."

He talked for ten minutes. About his older brother who had died in a hospice program in Lagos in 1998. About the way his brother had seemed to disappear in the last week, heavily sedated, barely able to speak. About how his sister in law had told him afterward that the medications had taken their brother away before the cancer did.

Elena said, "So when you think about hospice, what you see is your brother being taken away by the medicine before he was taken by the disease."

Mr. Afolabi said, "Yes."

Elena did not correct him. She did not explain that American hospice is different. She said, "That is a hard memory to carry. I understand now why you keep saying no. You do not want that to happen to you."

He said, "No. I want to be awake when I go."

Elena said, "Can I tell you a little about how pain management works now, not what it used to look like, but what it looks like in the hospice I know here. Would that be okay?"

He said yes.

She explained, briefly and without a sales pitch. She said many hospice patients are awake and able to talk in their last days. She said the goal is to match medication to the patient's preferences, not to sedate. She said some patients do prefer more sedation at the end, and that is their choice, but nobody forces it.

Mr. Afolabi asked if he could think about it.

He enrolled two weeks later. He died four weeks after that, in his own bed, with his children around him, awake for most of his final evening.

What this means for you: The reason Mr. Afolabi could not accept hospice from his oncologist was that the word meant "my brother." The oncologist never knew that, because he never asked. Once the meaning was named, it could be worked with. The key move was not persuasion. It was asking what hospice meant to him, accepting the answer, and offering information only when he asked for it.

10.7 Another Real Example

Meet David. He was a home hospice medical director in rural Tennessee. His team had been getting referrals from a local pulmonologist whose patients kept declining hospice. The referral rate was fine. The enrollment rate was terrible.

David called the pulmonologist and asked if he could ride along on a clinic day. The pulmonologist, a tired man named Raj, agreed.

David watched Raj talk to four patients in one afternoon. Raj was competent, caring, and direct. With each patient who had end stage COPD, Raj said some version of: "Your lungs are getting worse. I think it is time for hospice. Hospice will keep you comfortable. Are you willing to sign up?"

Each patient, with some variation, said no. Raj accepted the no and moved on.

In the car afterward, David asked Raj what Raj thought the patients had heard.

Raj said, "That I thought they were dying and it was time to stop trying."

David said, "Yes."

They talked about what else Raj might say. David described the "layer" frame. He suggested Raj start by asking what the patient understood about their COPD, then what mattered to them, then what hospice might add, rather than what it meant.

Raj tried it the next week. He called David two weeks after that and said three of five patients he had talked with had enrolled. The patients were the same. The disease stage was the same. What had changed was how Raj opened the conversation.

What this means for you: The hospice conversation is not a solo performance by a single clinician. It is often improved by coaching between team members. If you are a palliative care nurse, physician, or social worker, part of your job is to help the colleagues who refer to you get better at the conversation that precedes the referral. That coaching can do more good for more patients than your direct work with any one family.

10.8 When It Does Not Work

The most common failure is that the clinician keeps pushing after the patient has said no the first time. The clinician has a list of benefits. They produce them one after another. The patient produces a new reason for no after each benefit. The clinician fights the list with the list. The conversation ends with both sides exhausted and the patient less likely to say yes next time than they would have been before the conversation started.

Three things to try when you hit a wall:

1. When you feel yourself starting to list benefits, stop. Ask a question instead. "Help me understand what concerns you most about this." The conversation returns to the patient's frame. 2. When the no is firm, accept it. Say, "You are not ready for this today. Can we just set this aside and talk about something else? We can come back to it when you want to." Real acceptance is the most powerful thing you can offer, because it is rare. 3. If you cannot hold yourself back from pushing, it may be that you care too much about the outcome for the conversation to work. Sometimes the best move is to ask a colleague to take the next hospice conversation with that patient. There is no shame in recognizing that your own attachment is in the way.

A second failure mode is rushing the pre work. You ask about values and understanding, but you race through those questions to get to hospice. The patient feels the rushing. They know you have an agenda. They respond to the agenda rather than the conversation. If you only have time to do the pre work properly or only time to mention hospice, do the pre work. The hospice conversation can wait.

10.9 The Quick Version

Hospice is not a cliff. It is a layer. But the word hospice arrives in most patients' ears pre loaded with associations about endings, giving up, and imminent death. Before you mention the word, prepare the soil. Elicit values. Establish a shared picture of the illness. Ask what the patient already knows about hospice. The answer to that last question will tell you what file you are activating, and you can work with that file rather than against it.

When the patient says no, do not argue. Roll with the resistance. Ask what the no is made of. The fear underneath the no is usually what you can actually address. Common fears include sedation, losing a trusted doctor, insurance losing coverage, admitting to dying, or disappointing family. Each of these is a different conversation.

Accept the first no with grace. Many patients who eventually enroll say no at least once. The second and third conversations often matter more than the first. When you return, lead with how they are doing, not with hospice. Let them bring it up. If they do not, offer a gentle revisit without pressure.

Some patients never enroll. That is sometimes the right outcome for that patient. Your job is to make the door available, not to force anyone through it.

The next chapter goes into the most specific communication skill in this field: breaking bad news in a way that respects the person receiving it. It builds on everything in Part II and connects directly to the hospice conversation you just walked through.

Chapter 11: Breaking Bad News The Slow Way

Amara had been a clinical nurse specialist in cancer care for twenty six years. She had been in more bad news conversations than she could count. She was often the one physicians called when they wanted someone with experience in the room. At a regional palliative care conference in 2018, she was asked to give a talk on communication. She stood in front of two hundred nurses and doctors and said something that surprised them.

She said, "For the first nine years of my career, I thought breaking bad news was about finding the right words. For the last seventeen years, I have thought it was about how much time I leave around the words I say."

She told a story. In her tenth year, she had been in a room with a young mother, Gemma, whose breast cancer had spread to her liver. The oncologist had delivered the news efficiently. Gemma had listened, asked two questions, and left. Amara had walked her to the parking lot. In the parking lot, Gemma had collapsed to her knees and said, "I didn't hear anything after 'liver.'"

Amara had sat with her on the curb for forty minutes. Gemma told her everything she had not said in the exam room. When they went back in, the oncologist was gone. The conversation that had been held in eight minutes had not actually happened. The words had been said. The communication had not occurred.

Amara said to the conference audience, "The oncologist was a good doctor. He was kind. He had all the right words. What he did not have was time around the words. Bad news does not land when you say it. It lands in the silence you leave after you say it. If you do not leave that silence, the words bounce off."

This chapter is about what Amara learned in her tenth year. You will meet the discipline of pacing, the move of asking permission before sharing prognosis, the pause that feels too long, the practice of reflecting emotion before advancing content, and the closing that keeps the conversation open rather than sealing it.

11.1 Pacing

Most bad news conversations fail on pacing. The clinician delivers too many pieces of information too quickly. The patient catches the first sentence and loses the rest. What the clinician experiences as "giving a full picture" the patient experiences as being hit by a wave.

The discipline is to deliver one sentence at a time, then wait.

Compare two openings of the same conversation.

Version one: "The scans we did last week show that your cancer has spread to your liver and lungs. This changes the treatment options we have. Dr. Patel and I think it is time to consider stopping the chemotherapy, because the chemotherapy is not working and it is making you sick. We would like to talk about hospice and what your goals for the rest of your life might look like."

That is six pieces of information in four sentences. The patient has heard "spread to your liver and lungs." They are now processing that. Everything after it is gone.

Version two: "The scans show that the cancer has spread." Pause.

Wait.

The patient will respond. Maybe with a word. Maybe with a question. Maybe with a look at their spouse. You follow their lead. You do not move to the next sentence until the first one has landed.

Version two takes longer than version one. Version two produces actual communication. Version one produces words in the air that nobody actually received.

The research on this is consistent. Studies of oncology consultations show that patients remember very little of what was said after a bad news disclosure, with retention in some studies as low as 10 to 25 percent of factual information (Jansen et al., 2008). Slowing down does not fix this completely, but it helps enormously. Patients who experienced paced delivery, with pauses and acknowledgment of emotion, remembered more and reported better relationships with their clinicians afterward (Back et al., 2005).

Practical pacing looks like this. You deliver one sentence. You pause. You watch the patient's face. You let them speak first. If they do not speak, you wait. Only after you have received their response, whatever it is, do you consider delivering the next sentence. Some conversations that you thought would take ten minutes take forty. Some conversations that you feared would take forty take ten, because the patient guided the pace. Pacing means being led by the patient, not by your agenda.

11.2 Permission Before Prognosis

Before you share prognostic information, ask permission. This is a small move with large effects.

"I have information about what we are seeing on the scans. Would you like me to tell you what I see, or would you rather I wait and tell you another time?"

"Some people want to know everything the medical team is thinking. Others want more limited information. Which type of person are you?"

"I can tell you what I think is likely to happen over the next few months, if that would be helpful. Would that be helpful, or would it be more helpful to talk about something else?"

These questions do several things at once. They signal that the patient has a choice, which almost no other medical encounter has ever told them. They give the patient a moment to prepare emotionally for hard information. They produce useful data for you: a patient who says "please tell me" is in a different mental state than one who says "not today."

Some clinicians worry that asking permission gives the patient a way out of a necessary conversation. This is a misunderstanding. Most patients, when asked, want to know. A study of patients with advanced cancer found that 71 percent wanted a prognostic estimate, while only 17.6 percent recalled ever receiving one (Enzinger et al., 2015). The problem is not that patients do not want to know. The problem is that we are not asking and we are not telling.

The patients who say "not today" are telling you something important. They are not ready to absorb the information now, but they may be ready next week. Respect the "not today." Come back another time. If you force it, you will end up in an Amara in the parking lot situation, where the words were said but nothing was heard.

A note on cultural considerations. In some cultural contexts, the family may be the unit that receives information, not the patient directly. Asking permission in these settings can look like "who would you like me to share information with, and who would you like me to hold it from?" This is not a workaround of disclosure ethics. It is a recognition that autonomy includes the right to delegate how information flows. A patient who says "please tell my daughter and not me" has exercised autonomy. Your job is to honor that. Chapter 21.0 goes deeper into cultural dimensions of disclosure.

11.3 The Long Pause

After you deliver a piece of bad news, there is a pause. The pause will feel too long. It almost always is not too long.

The research on pause length in medical encounters is revealing. Clinicians tend to wait about one to two seconds after asking a question before they speak again (Beckman and Frankel, 1984; Marvel et al., 1999). The best estimate of how long most patients need to begin processing hard news is between seven and fifteen seconds, and sometimes much longer. The gap between what we do and what is needed is significant.

Here is what the long pause accomplishes. It gives the patient time to understand what they just heard. It gives the patient time to decide how to respond. It tells the patient that you are not rushing to the next thing. It creates space for emotion to emerge without the clinician immediately managing it.

The discipline of the long pause is almost entirely about tolerating your own discomfort. Silence in a room where someone just received bad news is uncomfortable. You feel you should do something. You feel you should say something. You feel you should offer a tissue or a reassurance. These urges are about your discomfort, not about the patient's need. Your job is to notice the urge and not act on it.

One practical tip. When you have just delivered a piece of hard information, count to ten silently before you say anything. The counting gives you something to do that prevents you from filling the silence. Often, before you get to ten, the patient will speak. Sometimes they will not, and you continue to count to twenty. Almost never does the patient need you to fill the silence for them. What they usually need is for you to hold the silence with them until they are ready.

The exception is when the patient is visibly spiraling, crying hard, or showing signs of a physical distress response. Then you can offer a brief acknowledgment: "Take your time." "This is a lot." "I am right here." These are not conversation fillers. They are signals that you are present. They are short. After them, you return to silence until the patient guides what happens next.

11.4 Reflection Before Advancing

After you have delivered a piece of bad news and allowed the pause, the move is almost always to reflect what you heard or saw, not to advance the conversation.

The patient says something. You reflect it.

"You are thinking about your kids right now."

"You are trying to figure out what this means for the trip you had planned."

"You did not want to hear that."

If the patient did not say anything but you saw something, you can reflect what you saw.

"I can see this is hitting hard."

"Your eyes just changed."

"You are somewhere else right now."

The purpose of reflection at this moment is to let the patient know you are tracking them and not racing to the next thing. It also gives the patient one more moment before you introduce any additional information. Each moment of reflection compounds. The patient is slowly catching up to what they just heard, and your reflections are keeping pace with them.

In MI terms, the volley in a bad news conversation should usually be: clinician gives information, clinician pauses, patient responds (verbally or nonverbally), clinician reflects, clinician pauses, patient responds again. You might exchange three or four reflections before the next piece of content comes into the conversation. This pattern is hard to maintain under time pressure. It is worth maintaining anyway.

Compare these two continuations after the statement "The scans show the cancer has spread."

Advancing: "Given the extent of progression, we need to talk about treatment options. Dr. Patel and I have been discussing if it makes sense to try a different chemotherapy agent or to consider more of a symptom focused approach."

Reflecting: "This is a lot to hear."

The advancing version drives the conversation forward into content the patient cannot currently absorb. The reflecting version slows down and meets the patient in the emotional weight of what they just learned. Advance too quickly and you lose the patient. Reflect first, advance later, and the patient comes with you when you do advance.

11.5 A Real Example

Meet Marcus. He was a palliative medicine physician in his fifth year at a cancer center in Atlanta. His patient was Mrs. Okonkwo, a 64 year old woman with ovarian cancer that had progressed on three lines of therapy.

Marcus had thirty minutes scheduled. Her husband was present.

Marcus opened by asking what they understood. Mrs. Okonkwo said she knew the cancer had been "acting up." Her husband said the oncologist had "mentioned the cancer being stubborn." Neither of them used the word "progression" or "incurable."

Marcus asked, "Would it be helpful to share with you what I see from the medical picture, or would you rather start somewhere else today?"

They both said yes, they wanted to know.

Marcus said, "The cancer is growing despite the treatments we have tried."

He paused. He counted to ten. Mrs. Okonkwo's husband took her hand.

Marcus continued, "That means the chemotherapy is not working the way we hoped."

He paused again. Mrs. Okonkwo said, "Okay."

Marcus reflected, "You are trying to take this in."

She said, "Yes."

A minute of silence followed. Marcus did not fill it. Mrs. Okonkwo eventually said, "Is there another chemotherapy we can try?"

Marcus said, "That is a question I can answer. Before I do, I want to ask you something first. When you think about the next few weeks and months, what is most important to you?"

Mrs. Okonkwo said, "I want to be at my granddaughter's naming ceremony in November."

Marcus said, "Tell me about the naming ceremony."

She talked for five minutes. The conversation that unfolded after that was about how to maximize her chances of making the ceremony. It included a discussion of if another chemotherapy made sense, but the discussion was framed around her goal, not around the abstract question of what to do next.

The whole visit took fifty minutes instead of thirty. The couple left with clarity about what mattered to them and a plan that reflected it. Marcus's next two patients waited longer than scheduled. Nobody complained, because the couple who left the exam room looked like they had just been actually seen.

What this means for you: Bad news conversations that honor pacing, permission, pause, and reflection take longer than bad news conversations that do not. They also do what the shorter ones fail to do: they produce communication rather than words. The extra minutes are not a cost of good practice. They are the practice itself.

11.6 Another Real Example

Meet Nicole. She was a palliative care social worker at a pediatric hospital. Her patient was Javier, a 9 year old boy with relapsed leukemia. His oncologist had just told his parents that the experimental trial had not worked and that curative treatment was no longer available.

The oncologist had delivered the news in about four minutes. The parents had sat in stunned silence. The oncologist had said he would give them time and left the room. Nicole stayed.

She did not explain anything new. She did not offer resources. She sat down in one of the two chairs next to the parents. She said, "I am not going to say anything for a while. I am just going to sit here. If you want to say something, I am listening. If you do not, that is okay."

Javier's mother, Yuki, cried silently for about seven minutes. His father, Kenji, stared at the wall. Nicole said nothing. After the seven minutes, Yuki said, "I need to tell him. I have to tell him."

Nicole reflected, "You are thinking about how to tell Javier."

Yuki said, "I don't know how."

Nicole said, "You do not have to do it today. We can talk about how, when you are ready."

Kenji said, "Can we go see him?"

Nicole said, "Of course. Let's go see him. We can talk about the rest later."

She walked with them to Javier's room. She left them alone with him. She came back two hours later. She did not bring up the telling question. She asked how they were doing. They talked about Javier's favorite foods. About the movie he wanted to watch that night. Normal things. Nicole did not force the big conversation. She let them hold what they had been given.

The conversation about telling Javier happened three days later. Nicole helped them plan it. It went as well as such conversations can go. Javier listened. He cried. He asked questions. His parents answered them. He died six weeks later with clarity about what was happening.

What this means for you: Sometimes the most important move after bad news is to stop talking entirely. Not every conversation needs to proceed to next steps in the same visit. Some families need hours or days before they can think about anything beyond what they just heard. Giving them that time is not abandonment. It is respect.

11.7 Closing Without Sealing

The final move in a bad news conversation is a close that does not seal.

A sealed close says: "We have talked through this. Here is the plan. Call me if you have questions." The patient walks out with a sense that the conversation is done. A week later, when the grief catches up with them, they have nothing to do with it except sit with it alone.

An unsealed close says: "There is a lot here to sit with. I will come back in two days. Between now and then, write down any questions that come to mind. Nothing is off limits. I will be thinking about you."

The difference is subtle and important. The sealed close closes a door. The unsealed close leaves the door open. Bad news does not finish landing in one visit. It finishes landing over days and weeks. The clinician who closes in a way that leaves the door open is signaling that they will be present across the arc of the landing, not just for the initial delivery.

Some specific closing moves that keep the door open:

"I want you to know this is not a one conversation thing. We will come back to it."

"I am sure more questions will come up once you have had some time with this. When they do, write them down. We will go through them next time."

"Before I go, I want to ask: is there anything you want to ask me that you have not yet asked?"

That last question, in particular, is powerful. It signals that you are not trying to rush out. It gives the patient one more chance to bring up the thing they have been holding back. Often they do not. Sometimes they do, and the thing they bring up is more important than anything else in the visit.

One more note. Before you leave, tell the patient specifically when you will see them next. Not "I will see you soon." A specific day. The specificity is a gift. It tells them that the care will continue on a schedule they can count on. It also prevents the common bad news aftermath in which the patient sits at home waiting for a phone call that never comes because nobody scheduled the next contact.

11.8 When It Does Not Work

The most common failure in bad news conversations is speed. The clinician, under time pressure or internal discomfort, races through the delivery. The patient does not catch most of it. The conversation ends on schedule. Nothing has actually been communicated.

Three things to try:

1. Before you walk into the room, block off twice the time you think you need. Tell your administrative support that this visit is not to be interrupted. If you truly do not have the time on a given day, reschedule the conversation. Delivering bad news in a hurry is worse than delivering it two days late. 2. During the visit, watch the patient's face more than the chart. The face tells you if they are still with you. If the face has gone blank, you are past the point where new information is landing. Stop delivering. Reflect. Wait. 3. At the end of the visit, before you leave, ask the patient to tell you in their own words what they heard. Not what the plan is. What they heard. This diagnostic question will tell you if anything landed. If what they say does not match what you said, you have useful information about what to address next time.

A second failure mode is emotional distance. Some clinicians, trained to be professional, become remote when the stakes rise. The patient experiences this as abandonment. Presence does not require you to cry, but it does require you to be emotionally in the room. If you are intellectually organized and emotionally absent, the patient will feel it. The fix is not to perform emotion. It is to let yourself feel what is happening. A moment of honest feeling, shown on your face, is more supportive than any script.

11.9 What To Take Away

Breaking bad news well is mostly about time, not words. Pacing means delivering one sentence and waiting before the next. Permission means asking the patient if they want to receive prognostic information before you give it. Pause means leaving seven to fifteen seconds of silence after hard information, long enough to feel uncomfortable, and not filling it. Reflection means meeting the patient's response with acknowledgment rather than advancing to content.

Closing without sealing means leaving the conversation open rather than wrapped up. Bad news does not finish landing in one visit. It finishes landing over days and weeks. Your job is to be present across that arc, which means scheduling a specific next visit before you leave and signaling that more questions are welcome.

The most common failure is rushing. Block off twice the time you think you need. Watch the patient's face. Ask them at the end to tell you in their own words what they heard. If the answer does not match what you said, you know what to come back to.

The next chapter builds directly on this one. Prognosis is the hardest piece of bad news to deliver well, because the underlying uncertainty makes every clinician want to fudge. Chapter 12.0 is about how to talk about prognosis honestly when you are humbled by how often you have been wrong.

Chapter 12: Prognosis Without The Crystal Ball

Dr. Omar Farooq had been a palliative medicine physician for fourteen years. He taught fellows at a large academic medical center in Philadelphia. Every summer, as the new fellows arrived, he did an exercise that unnerved them.

He gave each fellow a list of the patients Omar had personally followed in the previous year. For each patient, the list contained Omar's original prognostic estimate (what he had predicted at the time of first consult) and the patient's actual survival. He asked the fellows to calculate his accuracy.

The first time he did this, in 2011, he had been personally shaken by the results. He had been accurate (within a third of the actual survival) on 38 percent of his cases. He had overestimated survival on 51 percent and underestimated on 11 percent. When he adjusted the accuracy window to "within half of actual," his accuracy went up, but the direction of error stayed the same. He was, like most clinicians, systematically too optimistic.

The fellows, hearing this, would ask if they should trust his prognostic opinions. Omar would say, "You should trust them as one input. You should not trust them as a verdict. The data is clear: we are not very good at this. The difference between a good prognosticator and a bad one is not accuracy. It is honesty about the limits of accuracy."

Then he would say something that became the orienting sentence for his teaching: "Prognostic humility is not a soft virtue. It is the foundation of honest prognostic conversations. The clinicians who are certain are the ones who get it wrong. The clinicians who know they might be wrong are the ones who can have these conversations without damaging the person in front of them."

This chapter is about that kind of prognostic work. You will see why clinicians overestimate survival, how to share prognostic information honestly without crushing hope, how to use the dual frame of "hope for the best, prepare for the worst," what to do when a patient says they do not want to know, and how to revisit prognosis when the clinical picture changes.

12.1 Why Clinicians Overestimate

The research on prognostic accuracy in terminally ill patients is humbling. The landmark study by Christakis and Lamont (2000) followed 468 patients referred to hospice in Chicago. The 343 referring physicians had given a survival estimate for each patient at the time of referral. The actual median survival was 24 days. Only 20 percent of the physicians' predictions were within a third of actual survival. Sixty three percent were overoptimistic. Overall, physicians overestimated survival by a factor of 5.3.

Read that again. Physicians referring to hospice overestimated survival by more than five times on average. Hospice referrals are already a population where clinicians have recognized the terminal state. Even at that point, we are mostly predicting too long.

Several mechanisms contribute. First, we are trained as optimists. Medical education emphasizes hope, intervention, and possibility. Pessimism in medicine feels like professional failure, even when pessimism would be accurate. Second, we see outliers. Every oncologist remembers the patient who was "given six months" and lived seven years. Those memories are vivid and atypical. They shape our intuitions toward longer survival estimates. Third, the longer we know a patient, the more optimistic we become. Christakis found that physicians who knew their patients longer made worse predictions than those who knew them less well, likely because emotional attachment distorts estimation (Christakis, 1999).

Fourth, clinicians confuse "best case" with "most likely case." When asked "how long does this patient have," many clinicians report a number that reflects their best case rather than their median expectation. The patient then hears the best case and anchors on it. When the actual outcome is closer to median, the patient feels betrayed.

The practical implication is that your prognostic sense, honestly examined, is probably too long. This does not mean you should swing to the other extreme and forecast doom. It means you should calibrate. When you find yourself saying "months to a year," consider if "weeks to months" might be closer to the middle of your distribution.

Better still, use tools. Palliative Performance Scale, Palliative Prognostic Score, and similar validated instruments are more accurate than clinician intuition in many settings (Glare et al., 2003). They are not perfect. They are usually better than you alone.

12.2 Honest Without Brutal

Honest prognostic language does not mean numeric precision. It means accurate communication of uncertainty, direction, and order of magnitude.

Consider three ways to share a prognostic estimate for a patient you believe has weeks to months to live.

Brutal: "You have four to six weeks to live." Dishonest: "It is hard to say. Everyone is different." Honest: "Based on what I am seeing, I think we are in the range of weeks to a few months. I could be wrong in either direction, but that is my best sense."

The brutal version pretends precision you do not have. It also lands like a sentence. The dishonest version dodges the question in a way that feels comforting but provides nothing usable. The honest version names a range, acknowledges uncertainty, and gives the patient enough to work with.

One useful structure is the "two weeks, two months, two seasons" framing. Rather than giving precise numbers, you orient the patient within an order of magnitude. "You are not in the two week range. You are in the two month range, maybe a bit longer, maybe a bit shorter." This language is easier for patients to work with than specific numbers, and it is more honest about what you actually know.

When asked directly ("how long do I have"), a useful response is: "I wish I could give you a better answer than I can. What I can tell you is what I am seeing. I think we are in [orient to range]. I have been wrong in both directions for many patients. Some people surprise us by lasting longer. Some get sicker faster than we expect. If you tell me what you would do differently with the information, I can help you make the most of it."

The last move in that sentence is important. The patient is asking for a number because they want to do something with the number. If you ask what they would do differently, you get to the thing underneath the question. A patient who wants to plan a trip in two months needs to know if two months is reasonable. A patient who wants to make financial arrangements needs to know what the order of magnitude is. A patient who wants to tell their children needs to know how urgent the telling is. Once you know what they are trying to do, you can help them plan without pretending to know the unknowable.

12.3 Hope And Prepare

One of the most useful frames in palliative communication is the dual frame sometimes called "hope for the best, prepare for the worst" (Back et al., 2003). The idea is that you invite the patient to hold two things at once: active hope for better outcomes and active preparation for worse ones.

In practice, this sounds like:

"I want us to hope for the best and prepare for the worst at the same time. Is that something we can do together?"

"What does hope for the best look like for you right now? What would hoping for the best involve?"

"What does preparing for the worst look like? What would preparing involve?"

Note what this does. It does not force the patient to pick between hope and realism. It names them as parallel tracks that can both operate. It invites the patient to define each in their own terms. And it positions the clinician as partner in both, rather than someone trying to pull them from hope to realism.

The evidence suggests that this frame increases patient engagement with advance care planning without diminishing their sense of hope. A study of palliative care patients found that those whose clinicians used parallel framing completed advance directives at higher rates while reporting similar or better emotional wellbeing than those whose clinicians focused only on worst case preparation (Jacobsen et al., 2018).

One phrase that works within this frame: "I hope your situation is different. I also want to make sure that if it is not, we have a plan that honors what is important to you." This sentence holds hope and realism side by side without asking the patient to choose.

A common concern about this frame is that clinicians worry they are encouraging false hope. They are not, if the "best case" they are hoping for is genuinely possible. A patient with metastatic pancreatic cancer hoping to beat the disease entirely is hoping against what the evidence supports. A patient hoping to make it to their daughter's graduation in four months is hoping for something that is possible in many cases, even if unlikely. The frame works when both tracks are honest. If you would not privately hope for the best case the patient has named, you need a different frame.

12.4 A Real Example

Meet Isabella. She was a palliative care NP at a community cancer center. Her patient was Mr. Park, a 68 year old man with stage IV non small cell lung cancer. He had completed two lines of therapy and was progressing. His oncologist had asked Isabella to help him think about next steps.

Mr. Park had one specific question. "How long do I have."

Isabella did not answer directly. She said, "Before I give you my best sense, can I ask what you would do with the answer?"

Mr. Park said, "My son is getting married in eight months. I want to be there. I need to know if I should fly him home to do it earlier."

Isabella said, "That is a specific question. Let me give you my specific best guess."

She paused. Then she said, "I think there is a real chance you could make eight months. There is also a real chance you could not. Based on the progression we are seeing, I would say eight months is possible but not the most likely outcome. If making the wedding matters this much to you, I would not count on August. I would talk to your son about if the family could move it up, or if he could do something earlier."

Mr. Park said, "Okay. What about four months. Could I make four months."

Isabella said, "Four months I think is more likely. I could be wrong in either direction, but if you are planning around four months, that feels closer to what I would plan around."

Mr. Park called his son that night. The family moved the wedding up to April. Mr. Park made it. He died six weeks after the wedding.

What this means for you: Prognostic honesty is not a number. It is a calibrated range plus a recognition of what the patient is trying to do. When you connect the information to what the patient is trying to plan, the answer becomes usable rather than abstract. Mr. Park did not need a number. He needed help making a decision.

12.5 When They Do Not Want To Know

Some patients do not want prognostic information. They will say so, if you ask. Honoring that request is an important part of respecting autonomy.

"Not today."

"My daughter needs that information. I do not want it."

"Just tell me what to do next. I don't want to think about timelines."

"I am afraid if you tell me, I will give up."

Each of these statements is telling you something different. The first is about timing. The second is about delegation. The third is about preferred engagement. The fourth is about the psychological effect the patient fears.

When a patient says they do not want to know, the move is not to try to convince them. It is to honor the request, understand what is underneath it, and leave a clear path for revisiting.

"I hear you. I will not push this. Is there anyone else you want me to share information with? Your daughter? Your spouse?"

"Not wanting to know now does not mean you cannot want to know later. If that changes, tell me, and I will be honest with you."

"Would it help if I told you I will let you know if there is something you specifically need to know to make a decision? Like if something time sensitive comes up. Otherwise, I will not bring it up."

These responses keep the clinician in an honest relationship with the patient without forcing information on them. They also establish a mechanism for updates if circumstances change.

One situation is worth special attention. When a family wants to withhold prognostic information from the patient (a common pattern in some cultural contexts), you need to ask the patient directly about their preferences before agreeing to the family's request. "Some people want to know everything. Some people prefer that I share information with their family and not directly with them. What works for you?" If the patient says they want the family to receive information, you honor that. If they say they want to know themselves, you honor that, even if the family prefers otherwise. The patient's expressed preference is the guide.

12.6 Another Real Example

Meet David. He was a hospice medical director in Minneapolis. His patient was Mr. Kowalski, a 79 year old man with end stage heart failure who had been on hospice for eleven weeks. David's original estimate at admission had been "weeks to a couple of months."

On week eleven, Mr. Kowalski was still alive. He was weaker. He was sleeping more. But he was still talking, eating small amounts, watching baseball with his grandson. His daughter Aisha called David one afternoon and said, "I thought he would have gone by now. Is something wrong?"

David said, "Prognosis is not a deadline. I was wrong about how long he had. I am glad I was wrong. He has been able to have more time with you than we expected."

Aisha said, "But now what. Does he not belong on hospice anymore? Are they going to kick him off?"

David said, "He still qualifies clinically. The hospice benefit is based on the disease trajectory, not on hitting a specific date. The fact that he has outlived my estimate does not disqualify him. I want to update you, though: he is still dying. He is still on the trajectory we discussed. I was off on timing. I was not off on direction."

Aisha was quiet. Then she said, "So this could go on for a while."

David said, "Maybe a while. Maybe not. Given what I am seeing this week, I think we are closer now. But I have been wrong once. I could be wrong again. What matters more than my estimate is how you want to use the time you have left with him."

Aisha said, "I want to bring my daughter home from college."

David said, "That is a good use of this time. Do it soon."

Mr. Kowalski died the following week. Aisha's daughter had arrived two days before.

What this means for you: Prognosis is not a one time announcement. It is an ongoing conversation. When your original estimate is wrong, the move is to say so honestly and update without defensiveness. Families can work with updates. What they cannot work with is a clinician who pretends the original estimate is still accurate when the evidence says otherwise.

12.7 Revisiting Prognosis

Every change in the clinical picture is an opportunity to revisit the prognostic conversation. This is one of the underused skills in palliative care. Many clinicians deliver a prognosis once and then never mention it again, even when the picture changes substantially in either direction.

Revisit when:

The patient has a significant decline (new symptom, new hospitalization, loss of function).

The patient has a surprising stability or improvement.

Enough time has passed that the picture is meaningfully different from when you last discussed it.

The patient is making plans that seem to assume a different prognosis than the one you think is most likely.

The revisit does not have to be dramatic. It often sounds like: "I want to come back to what we talked about a few weeks ago. My sense of where we are has changed. Can I share that with you?"

The key move is transparency about your updated thinking. If you now think things are progressing faster than you previously thought, say so. If you think things are stabilizing and your earlier estimate was too pessimistic, say that too. Both directions require honesty. Most clinicians are more willing to update toward "things are going slower than I thought" than toward "things are going faster than I thought," because the first feels like good news and the second feels like bad news. Both, however, are information the patient needs.

One phrase that tends to work for upward revision of severity: "I want to be honest with you about something. Based on what I am seeing this week, I think we may be moving faster than I previously estimated. I could be wrong again. But I did not want to wait to say it, because it might affect decisions you are making." Patients almost always respond well to this. They do not respond well to a clinician who pretends nothing has changed while the patient's body tells them otherwise.

12.8 When It Does Not Work

The most common failure in prognostic conversations is false precision. The clinician, pressed by the patient for a number, picks one. The patient takes the number as a verdict. When reality diverges from the verdict, trust breaks.

Three things to try:

1. When a patient asks for a specific number, resist the instinct to provide one. Offer a range. Acknowledge uncertainty. Name the direction of your likely error. "My best sense is weeks to months, and I have tended to be too optimistic in the past." 2. When you offer prognostic information, say it once and then ask what the patient is hearing. "What does that mean to you?" gets you inside their interpretation, which is often not what you intended. You can then correct misinterpretations before they calcify. 3. Write the prognostic conversation in your note with the exact language you used and the patient's reaction. When another clinician sees the patient, they can calibrate to what was actually said rather than guessing at what was meant.

A second failure is avoidance. Some clinicians, having no confidence in their prognostic skill, refuse to offer any estimate. This leaves patients in a worse position than a calibrated range would. The honest move is to offer what you have while naming what you do not have. "I am not sure" is better than no answer at all, if accompanied by "here is my best range."

12.9 Where You Are Now

Prognostic humility is the precondition for honest prognostic work. Clinicians overestimate survival by large factors in most studies. The clinicians who know this and account for it do better than those who believe they are accurate. The best move is to calibrate downward in most cases, use validated tools when available, and communicate ranges rather than numbers.

The dual frame of hoping for the best while preparing for the worst holds both tracks open without making the patient choose. The patient's autonomy to decline prognostic information is real, and you honor it by asking about preferences, offering alternatives (like delegating to a family member), and leaving the door open for later engagement.

Every change in the clinical picture is a reason to revisit the prognosis. Update honestly in either direction. Upward revisions of severity are harder to deliver but essential when the picture has changed.

The next chapter turns to what happens after the prognosis has been discussed. Goals of care conversations build on the prognostic foundation. They ask what the patient wants their remaining time to look like. Chapter 13.0 is about how to run those conversations so the resulting goals actually hold as the situation evolves.

Chapter 13: Goals Of Care That Hold

On Tuesday morning, Marcus, a palliative care physician, held a family meeting for Mrs. Petrova, a 74 year old woman with advanced COPD. The meeting went well. Her two children agreed to a plan of comfort focused care at home, no more hospital admissions, and a focus on being present with their mother. Marcus left the meeting feeling pleased. The plan was clear. Everyone was aligned. He charted it.

On Friday afternoon, Mrs. Petrova became acutely short of breath at home. Her daughter panicked and called 911. The paramedics intubated her on the scene and transferred her to the ED. She was admitted to the ICU. By Saturday morning, when Marcus got the consult note, she was on mechanical ventilation in an ICU bed, the exact outcome the family had agreed to avoid three days earlier.

Marcus went to the ICU. He found the daughter crying in the waiting room. She said, "I don't know what happened. I knew the plan. I just panicked. When I heard her trying to breathe, I couldn't do nothing."

The plan had collapsed not because the family rejected it. It had collapsed because it had been a plan about procedures (no intubation, no hospital, comfort at home) without being a plan about what to do when the moment arrived. The daughter had not had a script for the moment. She had the plan in her head. She did not have the plan in her hands.

This chapter is about what makes goals of care plans hold and what makes them collapse. You will learn why goals need to be expressions of values rather than lists of procedures. You will meet the distinction between concordance and consensus. You will see why "what do you want us to do" is the wrong opening question.

You will learn how to hold the goals through the medical storm, and how to renegotiate them when the body changes.

13.1 Goals As Values

A goals of care plan that lives only as a list of procedures will not hold. "No intubation, no CPR, no transfer to hospital" is a specification of what not to do. In the moment, when the phone rings at 2 a.m. and the patient is gasping, the family member needs more than a specification. They need to know why.

When the plan is connected to values, the "why" is built in. "We want her at home because she has said many times that she wants to die at home" is a values statement. The procedures fall out of it. "No intubation" means "no intubation because she does not want to die on a ventilator." The procedure is downstream of the value.

When the family member faces the moment, the values are what travels with them. The daughter who hears her mother gasping and knows that "mom wanted to die at home" can breathe through the panic and call the hospice line rather than 911. The daughter who only knows "no hospital" but does not have the value behind it will panic and call 911, because in the moment "no hospital" does not feel strong enough to withstand the fear.

The translation is crucial. A goals of care conversation should produce:

The values the patient holds about the end of life.

The decisions those values support.

The plan for specific moments when those decisions will be tested.

Most goals of care conversations produce only the second of these three. They generate lists of preferences, often in the form of a POLST or an advance directive. Those lists are necessary but not sufficient. Without the values underneath and the specific plans around them, the preferences do not hold under stress.

13.2 Concordance Not Consensus

Concordance is the alignment of care with the patient's values. **Consensus** is when everyone in the room agrees. These are not the same thing, and families often conflate them, which is one reason goals of care meetings collapse.

Consensus is a goal many clinicians pursue because it feels clean. Everyone nods. Everyone agrees. The document gets signed. The problem is that consensus can be achieved by people agreeing out loud to things they do not actually believe. A son who disagrees with the plan may nod because he does not want to fight in front of his dying father. That nod does not mean he will support the plan when the crisis comes. It means he is uncomfortable disagreeing in a family meeting.

Concordance is different. It is not about everyone agreeing. It is about the plan reflecting the patient's own values. The family does not have to all personally prefer the plan. They have to understand that it is the patient's own values driving it.

In practice, this means the facilitator of a goals of care meeting is not trying to bring the family to agreement. The facilitator is trying to help the family see what the patient's values are, and then to plan based on those values.

This shows up in specific language. Compare these two kinds of questions:

Consensus question: "Does everyone agree we should stop aggressive treatment?"

Concordance question: "Given what your mother has said mattered to her, what do we think she would want us to do?"

The first question asks the family to decide. The second question asks the family to discern. These are different cognitive tasks. Deciding requires the family members to weigh their own preferences. Discerning requires them to look together at their mother's values and figure out what those values point to.

Families are often more able to discern than to decide. A son who cannot bring himself to "agree" to stopping treatment may be able to say "I know she would not want this." The statement reflects the same conclusion but through a different path. The path matters, because the path is what survives the emotional storm when the decision point arrives.

13.3 Not "What Do You Want Us To Do"

One of the most common opening moves in a goals of care meeting is a disaster. "What do you want us to do?" The clinician means well. The family hears something specific: "you have to make a decision about your dying mother right now with no information."

The question puts the entire burden of deciding on the family. It positions the clinician as an order taker rather than a partner. It also produces bad answers. Families under pressure, asked to make big decisions, often pick the most aggressive option because it feels like "doing something." They may regret it later. They will certainly not own it in a way that holds.

Better openings position the conversation as collaborative and start with understanding rather than deciding.

"Before we talk about what to do, I want to make sure we are all on the same page about what is happening. Can I share what I am seeing medically, and then we can talk together about what that means?"

"I want to understand what is most important to your mother, and what is most important to each of you, before we talk about specific choices. Can we start there?"

"This is a decision we should make together. I have some medical expertise. You have expertise about your mother. Let's combine what we each know."

These openings do several things. They slow down the rush to decision. They position the clinician as partner. They acknowledge that the family has expertise. They set up the conversation to produce concordance, not just a signed form.

The REMAP framework from Childers and colleagues (2017) formalizes this approach. REMAP stands for Reframe, Expect emotion, Map out values, Align with values, Plan. Notice that "plan" is the last step. The four steps before it are about building the foundation on which a plan can be made. Most goals of care meetings skip to plan. REMAP and similar structures insist that you do the foundation work first.

13.4 Holding Through The Storm

A plan made on Tuesday faces a test on Friday. The test is what clinicians sometimes call "the medical storm": the moment when a symptom crisis or an unexpected decline pushes everyone in the family out of the careful thinking they did in the calm meeting.

The goal of the calm meeting is to produce something that survives the storm. This requires three things beyond the plan itself.

First, a rehearsal of the moment. Before you leave the family meeting, ask: "What will it look like if Mom becomes acutely short of breath at home? Who will you call? What will you say? What will you do first?" Walk through it. Make the plan tangible. If the family cannot describe what they will do in the moment, the plan is not ready. If they can describe it, the plan is more likely to hold.

Second, a plan for the family's emotional response. Ask: "What do you think will be hardest about the moment when it comes? How will you feel? What will you want to do that might be different from the plan?" This opens a conversation about the daughter's impulse to call 911. Once the impulse is named, it can be planned for. "When you feel that impulse, call the hospice line instead. The hospice line is 800-xxx-xxxx. Put it in your phone now."

Third, a point person. Identify one family member who will be responsible for holding the plan in the moment. This is usually, but not always, the primary caregiver or the healthcare proxy. That person knows their job is not to make the decision in the moment. It is to enact the decision that was already made. This reduces the burden in the crisis from "what should we do" to "what did we decide to do."

The last piece is the most overlooked. Clinicians often assume that a family that has agreed to a plan will execute it. They often cannot, because they have not rehearsed, they have not named the emotional response, and no one person has taken ownership of the execution. Adding these three elements at the end of the goals of care meeting is a thirty minute investment that can save families from the collapse Mrs. Petrova's family went through.

13.5 A Real Example

Meet Yuki. She was a hospice social worker in her fourth year. Her patient was Mr. Oduya, an 81 year old man with advanced dementia, living at home with his wife and daughter as co caregivers. The family had done an initial goals of care conversation and had agreed to comfort focused care, no hospital transfers.

Yuki came for a follow up visit two weeks later. She did not ask if they remembered the plan. She asked, "If Mr. Oduya became acutely short of breath tonight, walk me through what you would do."

The daughter said, "I would call 911, because I would not know what else to do."

The wife said, "You would not. We agreed we would call hospice."

They started arguing.

Yuki said, "Let me stop you. This is important that we have clarified before it happens. Let's talk through it now."

She spent the next forty minutes helping them build a specific protocol. Who would call first. What they would say. What the hospice nurse would do. What the family would do while waiting for the nurse. What would happen if Mr. Oduya seemed to be dying. What they could expect in the first hour after death. How to reach Yuki if they needed to.

She printed a one page document with the steps and the phone numbers. She put it on the refrigerator. She made sure each family member had it in their phone.

Three weeks later, Mr. Oduya had a symptom crisis at 11 p.m. The wife called the hospice on call nurse. The nurse walked them through medication administration over the phone. The nurse came out within forty minutes. Mr. Oduya's symptoms were controlled. He died two days later at home, which was where he wanted to be.

What this means for you: The difference between a plan that holds and a plan that collapses is usually if the family has rehearsed the moment. Abstract plans collapse under pressure. Specific, step by step plans for specific situations survive. Your job is not to leave the family with the plan. It is to leave them with the plan and the rehearsal.

13.6 Another Real Example

Meet Raj. He was a palliative medicine physician at an academic medical center. His patient was Mrs. Laurent, a 62 year old woman with metastatic ovarian cancer. She had been engaged in goals of care conversations for several months. Her stated priority was "being clear headed enough to have conversations with my grandchildren."

Her disease progressed. Her bowel obstruction returned. The surgical team was considering another operation to relieve it. The surgery would likely extend her life by weeks but would require heavy sedation during recovery and might not leave her cognitively intact.

Raj brought this to her. He did not say "we should do the surgery" or "we should not." He said, "A surgery is on the table that might give you more time. It would cost you some clarity during recovery, and the clarity might not fully come back. When I think about what you have told me mattered most to you, the clarity seems to be the thing you valued most. I want to check: is that still true, or has your thinking shifted?"

Mrs. Laurent said, "It is still true. I would rather have three more weeks of being able to talk with my grandchildren than two more months of not."

The team supported her in declining the surgery. Her bowel obstruction was managed with comfort measures. She had three more weeks. She spent them with her grandchildren. She died at home, cognitively present, surrounded by the people who mattered most.

What this means for you: A goal is a decision criterion, not a single decision. When the medical picture changes, the original goal can guide the new decision if the clinician explicitly connects it. "Given what you told me mattered most, here is how I read this situation" is a move that lets the goal do its work in new circumstances.

13.7 Renegotiating

Sometimes the medical reality forces a renegotiation of goals. The patient who said "I want to keep fighting" six weeks ago is now weaker, sicker, and has to confront a question they did not face before. The facilitator's job at that point is to help the patient see that their goals may need to evolve.

The move is not to tell the patient their goals have changed. It is to invite them to look at their goals in light of the new reality.

"When we talked last month, you said fighting the cancer mattered more to you than anything else. I want to check in, because some things have changed. Is that still where you are, or has your thinking shifted as you have seen how things are going?"

"I hear you saying you still want to try. I want to make sure we are on the same page about what trying looks like now, because the options are different than they were. Can we look at them together?"

These openings do not impose a conclusion. They invite the patient to update their own goals in light of their own experience. Patients often do update, especially when given explicit permission. The permission is important because many patients feel they are not allowed to change their mind, that they are committed to the position they stated in the previous conversation. Telling them it is okay to update is often what lets them do it.

If the patient does not update and maintains a goal that the clinician thinks is unrealistic, the move is not to argue. It is to acknowledge the goal and work with its implications honestly. "I hear you still want to keep trying. Here is what trying would look like at this point, and here are the tradeoffs. Do you want to keep trying knowing those tradeoffs?" The patient gets to make the decision. The clinician gets to ensure it is made with accurate information.

Sometimes the renegotiation is one of location rather than aggressiveness. The patient who wanted to be home finds that home is no longer practical. The family is overwhelmed. The patient needs a level of nursing care that cannot be provided at home. The renegotiation is about inpatient hospice or a hospice house, not about changing the overall goal. The value ("I want to be as comfortable as possible with my family around me") can often be met in a different location than originally planned. Making the renegotiation about implementation rather than about goals is easier for everyone.

13.8 When It Does Not Work

The most common way goals of care plans collapse is Mrs. Petrova's situation. The plan was agreed to in the meeting. Nobody rehearsed it. The caregiver faced the moment alone and panicked.

Three things to try:

1. Never end a goals of care meeting without walking through the specific scenario the family is most likely to face. "What will you do if he becomes short of breath tonight?" Walk through it. If the family cannot describe it, they do not have a plan yet. Continue working on it. 2. Leave the family with a physical document. One page. Scenarios, decisions, phone numbers. On the fridge. In their phone. The document is an external reminder when the internal one fails. 3. Schedule a follow up visit within a week of the initial meeting. The purpose is specifically to test the plan. "Now that you have had some time, how does it feel? What has come up? What questions do you have?" Catching doubts early lets you address them before they become the reason the plan collapses.

A second failure is rigidity. The clinician, having done a careful goals of care meeting, treats the plan as fixed. When the patient's body changes, the clinician does not revisit. The plan becomes a relic of an earlier situation that no longer applies. The fix is to revisit proactively. Every significant change in the clinical picture is a reason to ask: given what we are seeing now, do the goals still fit, or do we need to think together about if they need to be updated.

13.9 The Main Ideas

Goals of care plans hold when they are expressions of values, not lists of procedures. The "why" behind the plan is what the caregiver needs in the moment of crisis. Without it, the procedures are too thin to withstand the fear.

Concordance, not consensus, is the goal of the family meeting. You are helping the family discern what the patient's values point to, not negotiating a compromise everyone can live with. This distinction changes the questions you ask and the way the meeting runs.

"What do you want us to do" is the wrong opening question. Better openings start with understanding, share the medical picture, elicit values, and only then move to plans. The REMAP framework formalizes this sequence.

Plans made in a calm meeting face a test in the medical storm. The test is survived when the family has rehearsed the moment, named their likely emotional reactions, and identified a point person to enact the plan. These three elements convert an abstract agreement into something that holds.

Renegotiate when the body renegotiates. Invite the patient to update their goals without telling them they have to. When the goal stays the same but the context changes, connect the old value to the new decision explicitly.

The next chapter tackles one of the most specific and loaded conversations in end of life care. Morphine and other feared medicines generate a particular kind of resistance from families.

Chapter 14.0 is about how to address those fears with the MI skills you have now built up.

Chapter 14: Morphine And Other Feared Medicines

Version one. A hospice nurse named Diego arrived at the home of Mrs. Abara at 10 p.m. on a Tuesday. The patient, Mr. Abara, 81, was in the last stages of lung cancer. He was actively dying. His breathing was labored. He was grimacing with every breath. Diego had instructed Mrs. Abara, earlier that day, to give her husband a dose of liquid morphine if his breathing became distressed. When Diego arrived, Mr. Abara had had no morphine in six hours.

Diego said, "Mrs. Abara, why haven't you given him the morphine?"

Mrs. Abara said, "I can't. It will kill him."

Diego said, "It will not kill him. The morphine helps his breathing. It is the right medicine for this situation. I need you to give him the dose now. He is suffering."

Mrs. Abara shook her head.

Diego said, "I understand you are scared. But I am telling you as a nurse, as a professional, the morphine is safe. If you do not give it, he will die in pain. Do you want that?"

Mrs. Abara started crying. She said, "Please. You give it to him. I can't."

Diego gave the morphine. Mr. Abara's breathing eased within twenty minutes. He died at 3 a.m. The next morning, Mrs. Abara told the hospice chaplain that she felt she had killed her husband. She carried that belief for the rest of her life. She would not let anyone speak of her husband's dying without her correcting them: "They gave him the medicine. He didn't just die."

Version two. Same home, same patient, same Diego. Different approach.

Diego sat down at the kitchen table. He said, "Tell me what you think the morphine will do."

Mrs. Abara said, "It will stop his breathing. That is what morphine does. My sister in law died of a morphine overdose. I know what it does."

Diego said, "You are afraid giving him this medicine will be the thing that takes him."

She said, "Yes."

Diego said, "I want to share what I know about how morphine works in this situation, because it is different from what happened to your sister in law. Is that okay to share?"

She nodded.

He spoke for two minutes. He explained that dosing for dying patients is calibrated to symptoms. He explained that his breathing was distressed right now because of the cancer, not because the morphine was missing. He explained that giving the dose would make the breathing easier for him without hastening his death. He explained that dying would happen if she gave it or not, because the cancer was doing that part, and her part was only choosing how comfortable he was during it.

Then he said, "This is your decision. I am not going to give the medicine unless you want me to. But I want you to know what I know."

Mrs. Abara was silent for a long time. Then she said, "You are sure it will not kill him."

Diego said, "The morphine will not kill him. His cancer is killing him. The morphine will let him be comfortable while it does."

She said, "I will give it."

She drew up the dose. She put it under his tongue. She held his hand. He relaxed within twenty minutes. He died at 3 a.m. She sat with him. She did not feel she had killed him. She felt she had helped him.

Both Mr. Abara got the morphine. Both Mr. Abara died on schedule from his cancer. The difference between the two versions is the difference between a widow who carried guilt for the rest of her life and a widow who knew she had done the last loving act her husband ever received.

This chapter is about that difference. You will learn the specific fears that drive medication refusal, how to assess health beliefs with open questions, how to use the elicit-provide-elicit structure for teaching, what to do when the fear is really about the death itself, and how to handle the midnight phone call when a caregiver is paralyzed.

14.1 The Specific Fears

Families refuse feared medicines for specific reasons, and the specifics matter. The most common fears are:

Addiction. "He will get hooked on it." This fear transfers from public health messaging about the opioid crisis, and it often comes from family history of substance use disorder. It misses that the pharmacology of end of life opioid use is different from the pharmacology of chronic pain management in a person with decades of life ahead.

Hastened death. "It will kill him." This is the fear that drove Mrs. Abara. It comes from media portrayals, family stories, and sometimes misinterpretation of what a clinician has said. It often rises when the patient is actively dying, because families connect the medication to the death that is happening.

Sedation. "She will be knocked out and we won't be able to talk to her anymore." This fear is especially strong when family members want to preserve conversation with the dying patient. It often reflects the family's grief about losing access to their loved one, not purely a fear about the medication.

Ceiling effect. "If we use it now, it won't work later when we really need it." This is the belief that opioids have a ceiling and that patients need to "save up" their tolerance. This is a misconception about opioid pharmacology in end of life care; opioids do not have a ceiling for most symptom management purposes, though they do require careful titration.

Moral concerns. "My religion says we shouldn't do anything to hasten death." This is often held by patients and families from religious traditions that have specific teachings about suffering, end of life care, or euthanasia. The worry here is often that pain management crosses a moral line.

Responsibility transfer. "If I give it, I am the one who did this." This is the fear that the person administering the medication will be morally implicated in any outcome. It is the fear that Mrs. Abara had most acutely, and it is often what is underneath the other fears when a family caregiver is the one being asked to give the dose.

Each of these is a different conversation. The response that addresses addiction ("in this setting, addiction is not a realistic concern") does not address hastened death ("the morphine will not be what kills him"). If you respond to the wrong fear, you will fail to reach the actual concern. The assessment of which fear you are dealing with must come before the response.

14.2 Assessing With Open Questions

The assessment move is a simple open question, asked before any teaching.

"Tell me what you think the morphine will do."

"What worries you about giving this medicine?"

"When you think about the morphine, what comes up for you?"

"What have you heard about morphine?"

Each of these invites the caregiver or patient to tell you what they are actually afraid of. The answer will tell you which fear you are dealing with. It will also tell you what personal or family history is driving the fear, which is often the piece that needs to be acknowledged before any information can land.

Common answers and what they usually mean:

"My uncle was addicted to painkillers" means the fear is about addiction, and there is a family history that the caregiver is bringing into this moment.

"I saw my mother die after they gave her morphine in the hospital" means the fear is about hastened death, and there is a traumatic memory associated with it.

"I want to be able to talk to her" means the fear is about sedation, and the underlying issue is the family's desire to preserve the relationship.

"The priest said morphine is okay for pain but not for hastening death" means the fear is moral, and the response will need to address the distinction between palliation and hastening.

"I just can't be the one to give it" means the fear is about responsibility transfer, and what the caregiver needs is not information but sometimes literally to be relieved of the act itself.

Knowing which fear you are dealing with changes everything about your response. A teaching moment about pharmacology will not help a caregiver whose fear is about responsibility transfer. An acknowledgment of moral concerns will not help a caregiver whose fear is about addiction. Getting the fear right is half the work.

14.3 Elicit Provide Elicit

Once you know what the fear is, the teaching move is **elicit-provide-elicit**, a structured way of sharing information that is fundamental to MI (Rollnick et al., 2022).

Elicit: You ask what the person already knows or believes.

Provide: You share information, briefly, with permission.

Elicit: You ask what they make of the information you just shared.

This structure has three advantages over straight teaching. First, it gives you information about what the person already believes, so you can target the teaching to what they need rather than what you assume they need. Second, it seeks permission before providing, which respects autonomy. Third, it checks for understanding afterward, so you know if the teaching landed.

Example, using Mrs. Abara:

Elicit: "Tell me what you think will happen if you give the morphine."

Provide (after permission): "I want to share what I know about how morphine works when someone is dying. Is that okay? [Yes.] Morphine in this setting is different from morphine given for other reasons. The doses we use are matched to what he needs for comfort. It will not hasten his death. The cancer is doing that on its own timeline. The morphine will help his breathing feel easier without changing how long he has."

Elicit: "What does that land as for you? Is that different from what you thought?"

Notice what the second elicit does. It does not assume the teaching was absorbed. It asks. The answer might be "yes, that changes things." It might be "I hear you but I still can't." Both answers are useful. If the caregiver still cannot, you now know the teaching alone will not do it, and you can move to the next appropriate intervention, which might be a direct nurse administration or a different kind of support.

The elicit-provide-elicit pattern is especially powerful with families because it creates genuine dialogue rather than one way teaching. Families often need to speak their fear, hear accurate information, and speak their response to the information, in that order, before they can act. Shortcutting the cycle usually fails.

14.4 A Real Example

Meet Aisha. She was a hospice chaplain in her sixth year. She had been asked to visit a family whose patriarch, Mr. Haddad, was dying of pancreatic cancer. He was actively dying. His daughter Fatima was the primary caregiver. The hospice nurse had reported that Fatima was refusing to give morphine even though her father was clearly in pain.

Aisha did not open with a teaching. She sat with Fatima and said, "Tell me what you are carrying."

Fatima said, "My sister and I were raised that we do not shorten life. Our father's imam has been very clear: you can treat pain, but you cannot do anything that hastens death. I don't know where the line is. I don't want to cross it."

Aisha was Christian, not Muslim, but she had worked with many Muslim families over the years. She said, "So the question for you is: is giving the morphine treating pain, which is allowed, or hastening death, which is not."

Fatima said, "Yes. That is the question."

Aisha said, "Would it help to talk to your father's imam together? I can call him if you would like. We can ask him this specific question in this specific situation."

Fatima said, "Yes. Please."

Aisha called the imam. He was available. The imam, Fatima, and Aisha had a conference on the phone for about twenty minutes. The imam explained his view: that morphine given to treat pain, even if it might theoretically hasten death as a side effect, was permitted under the principle of double effect, which is shared by Islamic, Catholic, and many other religious traditions. The intent was to relieve suffering, not to cause death.

Fatima cried. She said to the imam, "Are you sure."

He said, "I am sure. Give him the medicine. You are honoring him, not ending him."

Fatima gave the dose. Her father's breathing eased. She held his hand. He died about two hours later. She did not carry guilt about the dose.

What this means for you: Sometimes the fear you are dealing with is not medical. It is moral or religious. In those cases, the clinician alone may not be the right person to resolve it. Bringing in a religious leader, or another trusted voice, is sometimes the move that allows the caregiver to act. The clinician's job is to recognize what kind of fear is in the room and what kind of help will actually address it.

14.5 When The Fear Is The Death Itself

Sometimes the refusal of a medication is not really about the medication. It is about the death that the medication is associated with. The caregiver knows that giving the dose will happen in the last hours of the patient's life. Giving it feels like agreeing to the death. Not giving it feels like refusing to agree.

This is not a pharmacology problem. It is a grief problem.

When you sense that the real fear is about the death itself, the move is to acknowledge it directly.

"It feels like if you give this, you are agreeing to him dying."

"You are not refusing the medicine. You are refusing what is happening."

"You want to keep him here. The medicine feels like letting him go."

These reflections often open the caregiver to what they are actually wrestling with. Once the grief is named, it can be worked with. You can acknowledge that giving the dose does not cause the death. You can also acknowledge that the caregiver's instinct to hold on is love, not obstruction.

One move that helps in these situations is to rename what the caregiver is doing. "Giving this medicine is not agreeing to his death. His death is not yours to agree to or refuse. It is going to happen because of the cancer. What is yours to decide is how comfortable he is while it happens. You are not ending him. You are caring for him."

This rename is powerful because it returns agency to the caregiver in a way that is honest. The caregiver does not have power over the death itself. They have power over the comfort in the dying. Accepting that power is sometimes the hardest thing. Naming it clearly can be what allows them to use it.

If the caregiver still cannot act, the move is not to pressure them. It is to ask if they would like someone else to do it. "Would it help if I gave the dose? You do not have to. You are still his daughter. You are still loving him. You do not have to be the one to administer it." Many caregivers relax when they hear this. They did not realize they had the option. Once they know they have the option, they sometimes take it. Sometimes they say "no, I want to do it, now that I know I don't have to." The offering of the option is often what resolves the paralysis, whichever way they choose.

14.6 Another Real Example

Meet Marcus. He was a hospice nurse practitioner in rural Montana. He got a 2 a.m. call from a caregiver, Elena, whose mother was actively dying at home. Elena was supposed to give her mother a scheduled dose of morphine. She could not make herself do it.

Marcus was forty five minutes away. He could not be there quickly enough. He walked Elena through it on the phone.

He said, "Elena, tell me what is happening right now."

Elena said, "She is breathing funny. I am supposed to give her the medicine. I cannot pick up the bottle. I am just standing here."

Marcus said, "You are frozen."

Elena said, "Yes."

Marcus said, "What is the hardest part of the thought of giving it?"

Elena said, "If I give it and she dies, I will know I did that."

Marcus said, "You are afraid that giving the medicine will be the thing that kills her."

Elena said, "Yes."

Marcus said, "Elena, I need you to listen carefully. Your mother is dying because her body is shutting down, not because of anything you will do tonight. The medicine is not going to kill her. It is going to let her breathe easier. If you do not give it, she will still die. She will just die less comfortably. Does that make sense?"

Elena said, "Yes, but I still can't."

Marcus said, "You do not have to. Is there anyone else at the house?"

Elena said, "My brother."

Marcus said, "Call him in. Let him give it. This is not something you have to do. You can still be in the room. You can still hold her hand. You just do not have to be the one to administer the medicine."

Elena got her brother. Her brother gave the dose. Elena held her mother's hand until she died forty minutes later. Elena did not carry the paralyzing guilt she had feared, because she had not been the one to administer the dose. She had been the one who held the hand.

What this means for you: In the middle of the night, when a caregiver cannot act, the most helpful move is often to give them an option they did not know they had. The caregiver does not have to be the one to administer. The medicine needs to be given. It can be given by someone else. Relieving the caregiver of the specific act while keeping them present in the care is sometimes what allows the care to happen at all.

14.7 The Midnight Phone Call

Hospice nurses and on call physicians know the midnight phone call pattern. A caregiver is panicked. The patient is in distress. A decision needs to be made. The caregiver cannot make it.

The script for these calls, built from the work in this chapter, goes roughly like this:

Step one: Slow down the call. "I am here. Tell me what is happening."

Step two: Assess the fear. "What is the hardest part right now?"

Step three: Reflect what you hear. "You are terrified that if you give the dose, you are the one who ended him."

Step four: Share information, with permission. "I want to tell you what I know. Is that okay?" Short, accurate, targeted at the fear.

Step five: Offer options. "You can give the dose. You can have someone else at the house give it. If no one can, I can come out. What would be most helpful?"

Step six: Make a plan. "Let's decide together what you are going to do in the next ten minutes."

Step seven: Close without sealing. "Call me back in twenty minutes and let me know how it is going. If anything changes, call me right away."

This script is not rigid. It is a structure that keeps you from rushing past the emotional moment into the practical one. Most midnight calls fail because the clinician on the other end of the phone jumps to step four without doing steps one through three. The caregiver feels dismissed. The fear does not get addressed. The instruction does not get followed.

If you are the clinician getting these calls, practice the slowdown. Your first sentence after hearing what is happening should be an acknowledgment, not an instruction. "That sounds terrifying. I am here." Then assess what is underneath. Only then teach. Only then plan.

14.8 When It Does Not Work

The most common failure in medication refusal conversations is that the clinician treats it as a knowledge problem when it is actually an emotional or moral problem. The clinician explains the pharmacology. The caregiver still refuses. The clinician concludes the caregiver did not understand and explains again. The caregiver gets defensive. The cycle escalates.

Three things to try:

1. Before you teach anything, find out what the fear actually is. An open question ("what do you think the morphine will do") often reveals that the fear is not about what you assumed. Tailor your

teaching to the actual fear. 2. If teaching does not resolve the refusal after one round of elicit-provide-elicit, stop teaching. The barrier is not information. It is something else. Ask what else is in the way. "Even if the pharmacology were exactly as I described, what would still make this hard?" 3. Offer alternatives to the caregiver administering. Many caregivers freeze at the act, not at the decision. Letting them keep their decision making role while relieving them of the physical administration often resolves the paralysis.

A second common failure is moralizing. A clinician who is annoyed that the caregiver is "letting the patient suffer" communicates that annoyance, and the caregiver hears it as judgment. Whatever ability the caregiver had to act is further impaired by the shame. The work is to stay with compassion even when you disagree with what the caregiver is doing. They are not doing this to be difficult. They are doing it because they are terrified. Compassion is the only thing that can meet terror.

14.9 Pulling It Together

Medication refusal in end of life care is rarely about the medication. It is about the specific fears the caregiver brings into the moment: addiction, hastened death, sedation, ceiling effects, moral concerns, and the transfer of responsibility. Each fear requires a different response. Assessment with open questions tells you which fear you are dealing with before you respond.

Elicit-provide-elicit is the structure for sharing information. You ask what they already believe. You share information briefly, with permission. You ask what they make of it. This pattern is more effective than direct teaching because it creates dialogue rather than lecture.

When the fear is really about the death itself, the work is grief work, not pharmacology. Renaming what the caregiver is doing ("you are not agreeing to his death, you are agreeing to his comfort during it") can resolve paralysis. Offering the option of someone else administering the dose can free a stuck caregiver to take whatever role feels right to them.

The midnight phone call follows a structure that slows down before it teaches. Acknowledge, assess, reflect, share with permission, offer options, make a plan, close without sealing. The script is not a formula. It is a discipline against the instinct to jump to instruction before the emotional moment has been met.

The next and final chapter of Part III takes on the hardest conversations of all: stopping food, water, and treatment. These are the decisions that feel, to many families, like ending life rather than caring for it. Chapter 15.0 is about how to walk with families through those decisions without pushing them.

Chapter 15: Stopping Food, Water, And Treatment

You met Betty and Frank in Chapter 2.0. Betty was the 80 year old wife of Frank, who was dying of prostate cancer at home. Ellen, the social work intern, had met with Betty the day after Frank's nurse had told her that feeding him was now risky. Ellen had used a single reflection. Betty had cried. She had talked about sixty four years of meals. She had ended that visit saying she was not ready to stop feeding him, but she was ready to talk about it.

The next part of the story happened over the following three days.

On day two, Betty stopped offering Frank food and started offering him small sips of water. She told Ellen she had decided to keep the water because "water is not food." Ellen did not correct her. She sat on the couch and listened.

On day three, Frank started to aspirate on the water. He coughed. He could not clear it. Betty was terrified. She called the hospice nurse, who came out. The nurse did not tell Betty to stop giving water. The nurse asked Betty what she wanted to do.

Betty was quiet. Then she said, "I want to stop. I think he is telling me to stop."

The nurse showed her how to do mouth care. Swabs. Glycerin. Ice chips. Things that looked like offering without being offering. Betty spent the rest of Frank's dying using these. She did not feed him. She did not try to give him water. She dabbed his mouth every twenty minutes. She held his hand. She read to him from his favorite books.

Frank died on day five, with Betty holding his hand. She told Ellen at the bereavement visit that she had been terrified of stopping. She had felt that not feeding him was killing him. What changed her mind was not anything anyone said. It was Frank's body telling her what it needed. The clinicians helped by not pushing. They let her find her own yes.

This chapter is about the decisions that come up when food, water, or treatment are being reconsidered at end of life. You will learn what food and water mean to caregivers that the clinical literature does not fully capture. You will learn how to reflect the love beneath the offering. You will learn how to share medical facts without lecturing. You will meet the specific work of withdrawing mechanical ventilation. And you will see how to let a family find their own yes rather than producing it yourself.

15.1 What Food And Water Mean

Food is not food when someone is dying. It is sixty four years of meals. It is the last way the caregiver knows how to care. It is how the body is anchored to the living when everything else is slipping. For many caregivers, especially spouses and parents, giving food and water is the primary act of caregiving that has defined the relationship from the beginning. Refusing to continue it feels like refusing to love.

Clinicians sometimes approach the stopping conversation as if it is primarily about physiology. Tube feeding does not prolong life in advanced dementia. Forced fluids can cause edema and pulmonary congestion in the actively dying. These facts are true and relevant. They are not the whole picture. The whole picture includes what the food and water symbolize to the person offering them, and what their symbolic meaning has been across the course of the relationship.

The research on artificial nutrition and hydration in end of life care is clear. In advanced dementia, tube feeding does not extend survival or improve comfort (Finucane et al., 1999). In many terminally ill cancer patients in the last days of life, the effects of artificial hydration on comfort and symptoms are limited, and can include increased ascites, intestinal drainage, and secretions (Raijmakers et al., 2011). Dehydration at end of life can lead to a more peaceful death in many cases, with decreased need for catheters and fewer secretions (Heuberger, 2010).

But families are not mostly wrestling with the data. They are wrestling with what food and water have meant for the decades of life they have shared. A mother who has fed her child since birth does not experience "stopping tube feedings" as a clinical decision. She experiences it as stopping to mother.

The first move, before any discussion of medical facts, is to acknowledge what the act of feeding has meant. "You have been the one who has fed him for sixty four years. This is not just a medical decision for you. It is something else."

15.2 Reflecting The Love

When a caregiver resists stopping food or water, the resistance is usually an expression of love. Reflecting the love rather than arguing against the resistance is the move that creates space for movement.

Examples:

"Offering him water is one of the last things you can do for him. That is why you do not want to stop."

"You have fed him every day for sixty four years. Stopping feels like stopping being his wife."

"You are trying to keep her here through this. The food is the thing that has kept her here your whole life."

"The juice is not about the juice. It is about how much you love him."

Each of these reflections names what is underneath the behavior. The caregiver often responds with agreement and sometimes with tears. Both are useful. The reflection has made the love visible. Once the love is visible, the question of stopping becomes a different conversation. It is no longer "are you willing to let him die" (which the caregiver hears as the question). It is "how do you express the same love in a different way" (which is an answerable question).

The research on caregiver experience supports this. Families who felt their caregiving roles were seen and validated by the clinical team reported better adjustment and less guilt in bereavement than families who felt their caregiving was minimized or dismissed (Kramer et al., 2010). The clinical team member who names what the caregiver is doing, and why, is doing protective work for the caregiver's mental health after the patient dies.

One move that helps is to offer alternatives for the love to continue. If the caregiver cannot feed, they can still care. Mouth care with swabs. Reading aloud. Music. Hand holding. Lotion on the feet. Brushing hair. These are ways of expressing the same love in a form that is not harmful. Helping the caregiver see these as continuing acts of care, rather than as poor substitutes for "real" care, is part of what lets them stop the feeding without feeling they have stopped loving.

15.3 Facts Without Lecture

There is a place for medical facts in these conversations. The place is not at the beginning, and it is not ever delivered as a lecture. Facts work when they are offered with permission, kept short, and connected to the specific question the caregiver is wrestling with.

Elicit-provide-elicit applies here. You ask what the caregiver believes. You share information, briefly, with permission. You ask what they make of it. This is the same structure as in the morphine chapter, and it works for the same reasons.

An example, using Betty:

Elicit: "Tell me what you think would happen if you did not feed him today."

Provide (after permission): "I want to share what I know about what happens when people stop eating at this stage. Is that okay? [Yes.] What we often see is that people who have stopped wanting to eat are not suffering from hunger. The body at this stage does not need food the way it did before. Continuing to feed can sometimes cause more problems than stopping, because his body cannot process food well anymore, and the food can end up in his lungs."

Elicit: "What does that land as for you? Does that change how you are thinking about it?"

Notice what is missing from the provide. There is no "so you should stop." The conclusion is not handed to the caregiver. The information is offered. The caregiver decides what to do with it.

Specific pieces of information that often land well, when offered briefly and with permission:

Dying patients typically stop wanting food before they stop wanting water, and stopping wanting both is a normal part of the dying process, not a sign of suffering.

The sensation of hunger at end of life is often absent or diminished, and forced feeding does not relieve a sensation that is not there.

In advanced dementia, tube feeding does not extend life and does not reduce aspiration risk.

In the actively dying, fluids given by IV can cause swelling and congestion, while mouth care with swabs can relieve the sensation of thirst effectively.

Each of these is a short sentence of information. None of them is a full teaching on end of life nutrition. Caregivers do not need a full teaching. They need the specific piece of information that answers the specific question they are carrying. Your job is to know which one to offer, based on what you have elicited.

15.4 A Real Example

Meet Hassan. He was a hospice medical director in Arizona. His patient was Mr. Thornton, an 82 year old man with advanced dementia who had stopped eating six weeks ago. His family was split. His wife wanted to stop tube feedings. His daughter wanted to continue. The team had requested a family meeting.

Hassan did not open with a recommendation. He opened with a question. "Before we talk about what to do, I want to hear from each of you about what feeding has meant to your family."

The wife, Elena, talked about sixty one years of making him Sunday dinner. About how food had been how she showed love. About how she could still make the meals, even now, and her daughter could take them to the facility. Her voice broke.

The daughter, Aisha, talked about watching her father eat one of her mother's meals with pleasure two years ago. About how if they stopped the tube, she would lose that image. About how she was not ready for it to be the last meal.

Hassan reflected each of them. "For you, Elena, feeding has been how you loved him." Nod. "For you, Aisha, the tube is how you keep some piece of the father you knew." Nod.

Then Hassan said, "Can I share something about what we are seeing with your father right now?"

They said yes.

He said, "He has been on the tube feeding for ten weeks. He is losing weight. He has aspirated twice. His skin is breaking down. The tube feeding is not helping his body the way it would have two years ago. What is keeping him with us is not the food. It is his body's own slow pace. The food is not giving him strength anymore. It is sometimes causing him more problems."

Elena cried. Aisha said, "So what you are saying is he is not getting better from it."

Hassan said, "He is not getting better from it. And I think he is not going to."

Aisha sat for a long time. Then she said, "I don't want to keep doing something that isn't helping him."

Elena said, "I don't either."

Hassan said, "What I want to suggest is that we try something. We can stop the tube feedings and keep him as comfortable as we can. Your mother, you can still cook for him. You can bring his favorite meal in, and we can give him tiny tastes on a swab. That can be the comfort feeding that keeps the connection."

Elena said, "I would like that."

Aisha said, "Me too."

They stopped the tube feedings the next day. Elena brought in Mr. Thornton's favorite cornbread. She put a crumb on his lips. He licked it. She cried. He died five days later.

What this means for you: A decision to stop feeding does not have to mean the end of the love behind the feeding. When you help the family find a way for the love to continue, the technical decision becomes easier. The cornbread on the swab was not clinically significant. It was emotionally significant. Both of those things mattered.

15.5 Withdrawing Ventilation

The conversation about withdrawing mechanical ventilation is one of the most intense in palliative practice. The family is being asked to agree to a decision that will, within minutes to hours, result in the patient's death. The decision feels, to most families, like causing the death rather than allowing it.

The work is similar to the morphine and feeding conversations, with specific additions.

First, time. Withdrawing ventilation is rarely an emergency. The decision can almost always be given a day or more. Families who are rushed into it often regret it. Families who are given time to arrive at it often feel it was the right thing.

Second, information. Families need to know what they will see. Before withdrawal, walk them through what the next hours will look like. The ventilator will be removed. The patient may or may not breathe on their own. If they breathe, their breathing may be irregular. They may have noisy secretions. They will be given medications to ensure comfort. They may die within minutes. They may live for hours. Rarely, they live for days. The information is not to scare. It is to prepare. Families who know what to expect cope better than families who do not.

Third, presence. Ask the family how they want to be present. Some want to be at the bedside holding hands. Some want to be in the room but not immediately next to the patient. Some want to be down the hall. There is no right answer. Your job is to ask, not to instruct.

Fourth, after. Tell the family what happens after the patient dies. Does the family have time with the body. Who comes next. What do they need to do. Many families do not know. Telling them in advance reduces the panic of the moment.

Fifth, language. The language you use shapes how the family experiences the act. "We are going to withdraw the ventilator" centers the action. "We are going to let him breathe on his own" centers his body. "We are going to stop forcing his lungs to do what they cannot do anymore" centers the reality. Different phrasings work for different families. Ask, if you can, what language feels right to them.

A useful framing for many families: "We are not ending his life. His lungs are no longer able to do the job the machine has been doing for them. We are going to stop asking the machine to do what his body can no longer participate in. His body will do what it is going to do. We will keep him comfortable for whatever comes next."

15.6 Another Real Example

Meet Ravi. He was a palliative care physician at a large trauma center. His patient was a 34 year old man named Javier who had sustained a severe brain injury in a car accident three weeks earlier. He was on mechanical ventilation. The neurology team had determined that meaningful recovery was extremely unlikely. The family had been discussing the question of withdrawing the ventilator for a week.

The family was seven people. Javier's mother, his wife, three brothers, a sister, and a best friend. They were not aligned. The mother could not say yes. The wife had said yes but was devastated. The brothers were split. The friend was silent.

Ravi had been meeting with them for four days. He had not pushed. He had reflected. He had summarized. He had offered the dual frame of hoping and preparing. The family had moved, individually and at different paces.

On day five, the family was ready to decide but the mother still could not. Ravi sat with her alone for forty minutes. He asked her what was hardest. She said, "If I say yes, I am the one who ended my son. I cannot be the one."

Ravi said, "You do not have to be the one."

She looked at him.

He said, "You do not have to say yes. You can let the others decide. You can stay in the room. You can hold him. You do not have to be the one to sign off. The rest of the family can do that. You can be the mother who loved him until the end."

She cried. She said, "I can do that?"

Ravi said, "You can do that."

She went back to the family. She said to them, "I will not sign anything. But I will not fight you if you decide. I am going to be with him."

The wife signed the withdrawal consent. The brothers agreed. The sister agreed. They stood around Javier's bed. The respiratory therapist extubated him. Javier breathed on his own for about ninety minutes. He died without apparent distress, with his mother's hand on his forehead.

The mother said to Ravi afterward, "Thank you for letting me not be the one. I could not have lived with being the one. I could live with being there."

What this means for you: Not every family member has to make the decision. Different family members can play different roles, and acknowledging that is sometimes what lets the family move forward together. The mother who could not say yes was still able to be present. The wife who said yes was still able to lean on the mother's presence. Dividing the emotional labor can be what makes the decision possible.

15.7 Letting The Family Find Their Own Yes

The thread through all of these conversations is that the family's yes, when it comes, should be theirs. Not yours. Not one you produced through pressure or persuasion. Theirs.

This is hard when you can see that a continued intervention is causing harm. It is hard when you know that stopping is in the patient's best interest. It is hard when the family is taking longer than you think they should.

The discipline is to trust the family's timing. Most families arrive at the right decision if they are given time, information, and respect for what the decision means to them. The families who come to the decision on their own timing do better in bereavement than the families who are pushed into it. The research on prolonged grief and complicated bereavement suggests that feeling pressured into end of life decisions is a risk factor for worse grief outcomes, while feeling supported in making one's own decision is protective (Kramer et al., 2010; Wright et al., 2008).

Your job is not to make the decision happen. Your job is to create the conditions in which the family can make the decision. Those conditions include:

Enough time (do not rush unless medically necessary).

Accurate information (offered briefly, with permission, through elicit-provide-elicit).

Acknowledgment of meaning (reflecting the love underneath the resistance).

Alternatives that preserve caregiving in non harmful forms (mouth care, music, presence).

Permission to have different family members play different roles.

Space to change their mind (decisions can be revisited).

A clinician who provides these conditions and then waits is usually the clinician whose families arrive at the yes. A clinician who applies pressure is usually the clinician whose families resist until a crisis forces an outcome.

Betty found her own yes when Frank's body told her what it needed. The family in Chapter 15.5 found their yes over five days of work, with different members arriving at different times. The mother found her own role when Ravi gave her permission to not be the one who decided. All of these arrivals took time. All of them held.

15.8 When It Does Not Work

The most common failure in stopping conversations is that the clinician tries to talk the family into it. The clinician has the medical facts. The clinician knows what is best. The clinician presents the case. The family either capitulates (and regrets it) or resists (and feels attacked).

Three things to try:

1. Before you share a single medical fact, acknowledge what the feeding or the ventilation or the treatment has meant. "You have been trying to keep her alive because she has been your life." The acknowledgment has to come first, or the facts will land as argument. 2. When you do share information, keep it short and offer it with permission. A single short paragraph, followed by a question about what they make of it, is more effective than ten minutes of exhaustive teaching. 3. When the family is not yet ready, do not push. Ask when they want to come back to it. Schedule the follow up. Give them another day. They will often arrive at the decision on their own, in their own time, when the pressure to arrive immediately is off.

A second failure is treating all family members as if they are in the same place. They are almost never in the same place. The wife, the daughter, the son, and the brother are often on four different timelines and dealing with four different emotional landscapes. Meeting with each of them separately, at least briefly, often reveals differences that a group meeting flattens. A good meeting structure for these conversations often includes individual check ins before the joint meeting, so the facilitator knows what each person is carrying.

15.9 Closing Thoughts

Stopping food, water, and treatment are the decisions that feel, to most families, like causing rather than allowing death. The work of walking with them through these decisions is the work of helping them see that the love that drove the offering can continue in a different form, that the medical facts support their own instincts more than they might think, and that the family's own timing for arriving at the decision is to be honored rather than overridden.

What food and water mean to caregivers is almost always more than calories. They are the accumulated acts of care that have defined the relationship. Reflecting the love beneath the offering is the move that creates space for movement. Sharing medical facts only lands when the emotional ground has been prepared, and when the facts are offered briefly through elicit-provide-elicit rather than delivered as lecture.

Withdrawing ventilation is a specific version of the broader work, with particular needs for time, information about what the family will see, attention to how each member wants to be present, preparation for what happens after, and careful attention to the language used in the moment. Different family members can play different roles in the decision. Not everyone has to sign off for the decision to be made.

The final thread is the discipline of letting the family find their own yes. Your job is not to produce the decision. Your job is to create the conditions in which the decision can be arrived at. When you do this well, the family arrives at yes in their own time. When you do it poorly, they either capitulate with regret or resist until a crisis forces an outcome. The first option, the yes that is theirs, is protective of them in bereavement. The second is not.

With Part III complete, you have now been through the hardest conversations you will face in this work. Part IV moves to the broader work of family systems: family meetings, relatives who disagree, the absent relative who arrives late. The skills you have built in Parts I, II, and III all apply. The next three chapters give you the frameworks for using them when the room has more than two people in it.

PART IV: WORKING WITH FAMILIES

Chapter 16: Family Meetings That Heal

Ananya had been a palliative care nurse practitioner for nine years when she walked into conference room B on the fourth floor of the hospital and counted eleven people in the chairs. The patient, Mr. Rodriguez, was an 82 year old man with end stage heart failure and early dementia, currently on a ventilator in the medical ICU. He had been in the hospital for nineteen days.

The eleven people in the room were Mr. Rodriguez's wife, his six adult children, two of his grandchildren, his younger brother who had flown in from California, and a man who turned out to be the family's pastor. Nobody had told Ananya the pastor was coming. Nobody had told Ananya there would be eleven people. The original family meeting request had named three.

The ICU attending physician, Dr. Farouk, had already told Ananya in the hallway that he thought the family was going to fall apart. Two of the sons had been arguing loudly in the waiting room. One of the daughters was not speaking to another daughter. The wife, who was the healthcare proxy, had been crying for two days.

Ananya sat down. She did not start with the medical picture. She did not ask who wanted to speak first. She said, "Before we talk about anything else, I want to hear from each of you, one at a time, what you understand about what is happening with your husband and father right now. I want to start with you, Mrs. Rodriguez, and then we will go around the room. There are no wrong answers. You can say 'I don't know' and that is a real answer too."

Over the next twenty minutes, eleven people spoke. Some said almost nothing. Some spoke for three minutes. One son, the one Dr. Farouk had said was angriest, cried in the middle of his sentence and had to stop. Ananya reflected each person briefly. She did not correct anyone. She did not advance to the next person until the previous person had finished.

At the end of the round, Ananya said, "I want to say back to all of you what I heard. Each of you is sitting with something a little different. Some of you are watching him suffer and you want it to stop. Some of you are not ready for him to go. Some of you are worried about what this is doing to your mother. Some of you have questions about what is medically possible and what is not. All of these are real, and they are all going to be part of what we talk about."

By the end of the meeting, ninety minutes later, the family had arrived at a plan. They would withdraw the ventilator the following morning after his brother had a chance to say goodbye alone. There had not been a vote. There had not been a dissenting voice at the end. The consensus had emerged, because eleven people had each been heard in a room where most of them had been talking past each other for days.

This chapter is about the work of that ninety minutes. You will learn how to prepare the room, the agenda, and yourself before a family meeting. You will meet the move of opening with values instead of options. You will learn how to rotate reflections around a room with many voices. You will see when and how to name the elephant everyone is avoiding. And you will learn the close that produces concrete next steps rather than vague agreement.

16.1 Preparing Before You Walk In

The quality of a family meeting is mostly decided before it starts. The preparation work is about three things: the room, the agenda, and yourself.

The room. A family meeting needs enough chairs for everyone, arranged so that people can see each other's faces. If the patient is in the room, the clinicians should not stand over them. Sit at the patient's eye level. If the patient is not in the room, the chairs should be in a circle or a loose oval, not in rows facing the clinician. The physical setup signals the relational setup. A clinician sitting behind a desk with the family in chairs facing them signals hierarchy. A clinician in the circle signals partnership.

Time matters. Block sixty to ninety minutes for an initial family meeting. Shorter than sixty is rushing. Longer than ninety exhausts everyone. Tell administrative support you are not to be interrupted. Silence your phone. If other clinicians will join, coordinate arrival times so the family does not watch people file in and out.

The agenda. Before you walk in, know what the meeting needs to accomplish. A typical agenda has four parts: check on understanding, share medical picture, elicit values and concerns, develop a plan. You may not get through all four in one meeting. Knowing the four parts helps you recognize where you are.

Also decide in advance: who is the facilitator, and who is the content expert. These are often two different people. A nurse or social worker or chaplain facilitates the flow of the meeting. A physician carries the medical content. When the same person tries to do both, one of them usually suffers. If you are running the meeting as a single clinician, you will rotate between the two roles, and you should be explicit with yourself about which role you are in at any given moment.

Yourself. Before you walk in, check your own state. Are you rushed? Are you frustrated with this family from earlier interactions? Are you carrying bias about what the right decision is? Take sixty seconds in the hallway to notice what you are bringing into the room. The work you do with families is affected by what you bring. You cannot eliminate what you bring, but you can be aware of it, which is the first step toward not acting on it.

One more preparation move. If you can, call the primary caregiver or healthcare proxy the day before the meeting. A five minute call. "I want to make sure I know what is most important to you going into tomorrow. What are you hoping we can talk about?

What are you worried about?" This call does several things. It tells the proxy that you see them as the point person. It gives you advance information about what the meeting needs to handle. It sometimes surfaces issues that would have ambushed you in the room.

16.2 Opening With Values

The temptation in a family meeting is to start with medical content. The family expects you to update them. You have the information. The fastest way to get to decisions, it seems, is to give the information and ask what they want to do.

The fastest way actually fails. A meeting that opens with medical content puts the family in a reactive stance. They are processing information, not contributing. By the time the meeting moves to values and decisions, the emotional tone has already been set by the heaviness of what was shared. People are defending or pushing back, not reflecting.

A better opening starts with the family. Not with their decisions, not with their opinions about treatment, but with their understanding and their values.

"Before I share what I am seeing medically, I want to hear what you are understanding and what matters most to you. Can we start there?"

"I want to know a little about your husband, who he has been, what he has cared about. Before I talk about what is happening in his body, I want us to know who the person is we are trying to help."

"Let me start by hearing from each of you. What do you already know about how things are going? And what is most on your mind coming into this conversation?"

Each of these openings turns the first ten to twenty minutes of the meeting into a listening meeting. The family talks. The clinician reflects. By the time medical content arrives, the family has been heard, the clinician knows more about the system they are working with, and the room has the right relational foundation.

This approach is sometimes called **values first, facts second**. It is not that facts do not matter. They matter enormously. But facts offered into a room that has not first been heard land differently than facts offered after the family has been invited in. The same words have different effects depending on the ground they are delivered on.

One specific opening question that has served many clinicians well: "If your [father/mother/husband] could speak for himself right now, what do you think he would say about what he wants?" This question does three things at once. It centers the patient. It activates the family's memory of who the patient is. It shifts the frame from "what do you want" to "what does he want," which is easier for most families to answer honestly.

16.3 Rotating Reflections

In a meeting with multiple family members, the facilitator's job is to ensure every voice is heard, without the meeting fragmenting into side conversations. The move is **rotating reflections**: you go around the room, invite each person to speak, and reflect briefly after each one.

The rotation does several things. It signals that everyone will have a turn, which reduces the urgency some family members feel to jump in. It surfaces the range of views in the family before anyone tries to speak for the group. It tells the facilitator which family members are carrying which concerns, so later in the meeting, specific issues can be directed to specific people.

A rotation might sound like this.

"Mr. Davis, Sr., I want to start with you. Tell me what is going through your mind right now." He talks. You reflect: "You are holding a lot. You are worried about your wife, and you do not know what she would want." Move on.

"Aisha, let's hear from you next. What is on your mind?" She talks. You reflect: "You are thinking about your mother's pain, and about what your father can handle."

"Marcus. What about you?" He talks. You reflect.

Continue around the room. The reflections should be brief. Ten to fifteen seconds. The purpose is to signal that you heard, not to solve anything yet.

Sometimes a family member will pass. "I don't have anything to say." Respect the pass. Say, "Okay. If something comes up later, jump in." Do not push. Passes are often from people who need to hear others before they know what they think.

Sometimes a family member will monopolize the floor. Let them for two or three minutes, then gently bring it back. "I want to make sure I understand you, and I also want to hear from your sister. Let me say back what I heard from you, and then let's hear from her." This move closes the current person's turn without cutting them off, and moves the rotation forward.

One person in the family will often try to speak for the patient or for the group. "We have talked about this. My father wanted comfort care." This may be true. It also may be one family member projecting their own view onto the patient. Reflect what they said, then ask the room: "Does that match what the rest of you have heard from him?" This invites the family to confirm or contradict without challenging the speaker directly. The answer will tell you if the group actually shares the view or if the one speaker is out ahead.

16.4 Naming The Elephant

Most family meetings have an elephant in the room. Something nobody is saying. Often the elephant is obvious to the facilitator, because they have been around many meetings with similar shapes. The family may not name it because it feels too heavy, or because they have agreed implicitly not to.

Common elephants in end of life family meetings:

The patient is dying soon and nobody has said so out loud.

One family member believes another is motivated by inheritance or guilt rather than care.

A spouse or caregiver has been carrying the whole load and resents the relatives who have not helped.

A child has not been to visit in months and is now demanding to be consulted.

The patient expressed wishes years ago that the family has not been following.

Religious or cultural expectations are shaping decisions that nobody is explicitly discussing.

An old family wound is playing out in the current decisions.

The facilitator's job is to sense when the elephant is keeping the meeting from moving. Not every elephant needs to be named in every meeting. Some are best left alone. But when the meeting is circling the same topic without progress, or when tension is rising and nobody can explain why, the elephant is often in the way.

Naming an elephant requires care. You are saying the unsaid. You do it tentatively, with permission, and without blame.

"I am sensing that there might be something in the room that we are not talking about. I could be wrong. Can I say what I am sensing, and you can tell me if I am close?"

"I want to name something I am noticing, and I want to be careful about it. It feels to me like part of what is happening here is that you are not all on the same page about the fact that your father is dying. Is that part of what is going on?"

"I am going to take a risk. It seems like there is some history in this family that is affecting how people are feeling about this decision. I am not asking you to tell me about that history. I am asking if we could set it aside for the next ninety minutes, because the decision in front of you is about your mother, not about the history."

Each of these openings does the same thing. It names what is visible. It does not assume it is right. It invites the family to either confirm or correct. And it does not blame anyone for the elephant being there.

When the elephant is named and confirmed, the meeting often shifts. The family relaxes. They have been trying to navigate around the thing. Once it is out loud, they can navigate with it.

Sometimes naming the elephant produces more conflict, not less. If that happens, do not retreat. Reflect what is happening. "I can see that naming that made things more intense for a few of you. That is okay. Let's sit with it for a minute." The increased intensity is often the productive part. Conflict that surfaces can be addressed. Conflict that stays underground distorts every decision downstream.

16.5 A Real Example

Meet Marcus. He was a palliative care physician at a community hospital. His patient was a 68 year old woman named Mrs. Kowalski with metastatic lung cancer. She had been hospitalized for respiratory failure. The ICU team had asked Marcus to facilitate a family meeting because the family was, in the charge nurse's words, "not functional."

Eight family members arrived. Mrs. Kowalski's husband. Her four adult children. Two of her grandchildren who were adults. Her sister, who had flown in from Milwaukee.

Marcus opened with the rotation. He asked each person what they understood and what was on their mind. The husband spoke briefly and defeatedly. The oldest son spoke about wanting more information. The oldest daughter, Elena, was the one the charge nurse had flagged. She spoke for four minutes, with anger in her voice, about how the hospital was "not doing enough."

Marcus reflected Elena: "You are feeling like the medical system is failing your mother."

Elena said, "Yes. I am."

Marcus continued the rotation. By the time he had gone around the room, he had a sense of the elephant. It was not about the medical care. Elena was the only one still insisting on more aggressive treatment. The others, in varying degrees, had accepted that Mrs. Kowalski was dying.

Marcus did not confront Elena. He said, in the middle of the medical update section, "I want to check something with the group. It seems to me that most of the people here are, in their hearts, accepting that Mrs. Kowalski is dying, and trying to figure out what a good death looks like for her. Elena, you are in a different place. You are not ready for her to die. I want to name that, because I think it is shaping the meeting. Is that accurate?"

Elena cried. She said, "She was supposed to come to my daughter's wedding. That was four months ago. She missed it. I am not done being mad about it."

The rest of the family looked at her. The husband, who had been defeated all morning, reached over and took her hand. He said, "I know, mija. I was mad too."

The elephant was named. The meeting changed. Elena was not convinced in one conversation that it was time to let her mother go. But she was seen, and the rest of the family was freed from trying to navigate around her resistance without acknowledging it. Over the next three days, Elena arrived at her own yes, with her family supporting her rather than working around her.

What this means for you: Sometimes the blocker in a family meeting is one person's unresolved grief, and the whole family has been tiptoeing around it. Naming it, with care and without blame, can free the room. The naming does not solve the grief. It lets the grief be part of the conversation rather than the hidden driver of the conversation.

16.6 Another Real Example

Meet Isabella. She was a hospice social worker. Her patient was Mr. Abebe, an 88 year old man with end stage renal disease who had decided to stop dialysis. The decision was his own. He had capacity. He had been clear about what he wanted.

The family meeting was about implementation, not about the decision itself. But the meeting was not running well. The family had six people. Two of the adult children had agreed to his wishes. Two were silent. One grandson, Omar, kept asking questions that implied he did not believe Mr. Abebe really wanted this.

Isabella reflected each person briefly as they spoke. She did not push back on Omar. When the rotation was complete, she said, "Omar, I want to come back to you. I hear you asking a lot about if your grandfather really wants this. Can you tell me more about what is underneath those questions?"

Omar said, "He raised me. I lived with him for six years. I just don't want him to be making this decision because he feels like a burden."

Isabella said, "You are worried he is choosing this to protect all of you."

Omar said, "Yes."

Isabella said, "That is a question you can ask him directly. He is still able to talk. Would it help if you and he had a conversation about it, just the two of you, and you asked him?"

Omar said, "I didn't know if that was okay."

Isabella said, "It is more than okay. It might be the most important conversation he has this week."

Omar had that conversation that afternoon. His grandfather told him he was not dying to protect them. He was dying because he was ready. Omar came back to the meeting the next day and signed the paperwork.

What this means for you: Sometimes a family member's resistance in a meeting is really a question they have not yet been able to ask the patient. Helping them ask the question directly, rather than negotiating it through the family meeting, can resolve what looked like group conflict. The meeting does not have to do all the work. Sometimes the meeting's job is to name what conversations still need to happen outside of it.

16.7 Closing With Next Steps

Most family meetings fail to produce concrete next steps. The conversation happens. People feel heard. The family leaves, and within 24 hours, nobody is sure what was actually decided. This is not because family meetings are useless. It is because the close was too soft.

A strong close does four things. It summarizes what was decided and what was not. It assigns who is responsible for what. It sets a time for the next communication. And it names what the family should do if something changes between now and then.

A sample close:

"Let me summarize what I am taking away from this meeting. We agreed that Mrs. Rodriguez wants to go home on hospice. The plan is for her to be discharged tomorrow afternoon. Mr. Rodriguez, you and your daughter Ananya are going to be the primary caregivers. The rest of the family is going to coordinate visits so your mother has company but your father is not overwhelmed. I am going to make sure the hospice intake is arranged for tomorrow morning. The hospice nurse will call you in the afternoon. If any symptoms get harder to manage tonight or tomorrow morning, you call me directly at this number. Did I get any of that wrong, and is there anything we missed?"

Several things are happening in that paragraph. The decisions are named. The responsibilities are distributed. The timing is specific. The fallback plan is clear. The final question invites correction.

Then the facilitator writes the summary in the chart while the details are fresh. Not as a narrative. As a structured summary: goals, decisions, who is responsible, next communication point. This note will be what the next clinician reads when they arrive on the next shift. If the note is vague, the next clinician will have to reconstruct the meeting from scratch.

One more close element: the emotional close. Before you leave the room, acknowledge what the family has just done. "This was a hard meeting. You showed up for your mother. What you did together today was not easy, and I want you to know it mattered." This is not hollow praise. It is a specific recognition of the labor of the meeting. Families remember these sentences for years.

16.8 When It Does Not Work

The most common failure in family meetings is running out of time with nothing decided. The meeting was scheduled for sixty minutes. At minute fifty five, the family has shared a lot but no plan has emerged. The facilitator panics and tries to force a decision. The family agrees to something under pressure. Within a week, the plan collapses.

Three things to try:

1. If you are at minute forty five and you do not have a plan yet, do not try to produce one in the last fifteen. Instead, end the meeting at sixty minutes with a clear interim plan and a scheduled follow up. "We have done a lot of important work today. We have not yet reached a final decision. Here is what we are going to do in the next 48 hours. We will meet again on Thursday at 2 p.m." Families are usually relieved rather than frustrated by this. 2. If the meeting is dominated by one person, consider separate conversations. Not every person in the family has to be in every meeting. Sometimes the most productive move is to meet with the dominant voice alone, and then reconvene the group after. 3. If the meeting is fragmenting (side conversations, interruptions, people leaving and returning), pause. Name it. "I am noticing that we are having trouble staying together in this conversation. Can we take five minutes, let everyone get water, and come back with fresh attention?" The break itself often settles the room.

A second failure is overreaching. Trying to do too much in one meeting. A family meeting rarely needs to solve everything. Its job is usually to do one specific piece of work. Identify what that piece is before you walk in, and let the rest wait.

16.9 Pulling It Together

Family meetings are not magical. They are structured conversations that, when done well, produce outcomes that ad hoc hallway conversations cannot. The research on family meetings in palliative and ICU settings is mixed on some outcomes but consistent on one: families who receive well conducted meetings report more empathy from staff, less post traumatic stress, and better bereavement outcomes than families who do not (Curtis et al., 2016; Glajchen et al., 2022).

The preparation work is mostly invisible. The room, the agenda, your own state. Five minutes on each, before you walk in, will shape everything that follows. Opening with values and understanding, rather than with medical updates, turns the meeting from a briefing into a conversation. Rotating reflections around the room ensures every voice is heard, while brief reflections after each speaker signal that you are tracking.

Naming the elephant is sometimes the move that unlocks a stuck meeting. You do it with care, without blame, and with room for correction. When the elephant is really out, the meeting usually shifts. When the elephant stays hidden, the meeting circles.

Closing with concrete next steps is what prevents the meeting from evaporating once people leave the room. Name decisions, assign responsibilities, set the next check in, and leave a fallback plan for the hours between. Write the summary in the chart before you forget. Acknowledge what the family has just done.

The next chapter moves from the structure of the meeting to the specific challenge of managing disagreement within the family. When relatives disagree about end of life decisions, the MI skills from Parts I through III take on a particular shape. Chapter 17.0 is about working with those disagreements in a way that respects each family member without sacrificing the patient's own voice.

Chapter 17: When Relatives Disagree

Mr. Oduya was 74 years old and still lucid. He had advanced pancreatic cancer. He was on hospice at home. His two daughters, Layla and Gemma, were both at his bedside on a Sunday afternoon. He had been having more pain than usual that day.

Layla said, "Dad needs another dose of the liquid morphine. He is clearly in pain."

Gemma said, "He had a dose two hours ago. We are going to knock him out. I want to talk to him before he goes to sleep for good."

Layla said, "He is in pain right now. Look at his face."

Gemma said, "Of course he is in some pain. He has pancreatic cancer. We are not supposed to make him so comfortable that he cannot speak to us."

Layla said, "This is not about you and what you want."

Gemma said, "It is exactly about what I want, because I am here and I am his daughter too."

They kept going. Their voices rose. Mr. Oduya, who had been dozing, opened his eyes. He looked from Layla to Gemma and back. Neither of them noticed. He closed his eyes again. His face tightened. A tear ran down his cheek.

His hospice nurse, Amara, came into the room fifteen minutes later. Mr. Oduya was crying silently. The daughters were still arguing. Amara did something that changed the room in under a minute.

She said, "I am going to stop both of you. Your father is watching you fight, and it is hurting him. I want us to step out of this room together for ten minutes."

Layla started to protest. Amara said, "No. Your father is going to be okay for ten minutes. The three of us are going to go to the kitchen, and we are going to talk. And then we are going to come back in here and be together with your dad, whatever we decide."

They went to the kitchen. Amara said, "I need you to see what just happened in that room. Your father was crying while you were arguing about how to love him. Both of you love him. He knows that. He also cannot die peacefully if his last days are spent watching his daughters fight."

Both of them started crying.

Amara said, "I am not going to tell you who is right about the morphine. You are both right. He is in pain. He also wants to be able to talk to you. These are both true. We can work with both of these, but we cannot do it if you are fighting in front of him."

They worked out a plan. Small doses, more frequent, so he could have pain relief without being over sedated. They agreed on the plan together. They went back into the room. For the rest of that afternoon, and for the four days he had left, they did not fight in his presence. He died the following Thursday, with both daughters holding his hands.

This chapter is about that work. You will learn why family disagreement intensifies near death, how to reflect each perspective to the room, how to locate the shared value beneath the dispute, when the primary decision maker has to hold firm despite disagreement, and how to set clear limits on open conflict in the patient's presence.

17.1 Why Disagreement Intensifies

Relatives who have gotten along for decades often fight hard at the end of life. This is not about bad character or old grudges, though both can be involved. It is about what the situation does to people.

Understanding the mechanism helps you work with the disagreement rather than against it.

Several things are happening at once.

Grief is doing what grief does. Grief does not arrive neatly. It arrives as anger, as control, as blame, as numbness, and as desperation to keep the dying person here longer. Family members are often grieving at different rates and in different styles, which means they are emotionally in different places when they walk into the same room. Two siblings grieving differently can feel to each other like two people on different sides, when really they are on the same side at different stages.

Unfinished business is surfacing. Family systems carry decades of unspoken tensions. When one member is dying, everything that has been packed away comes loose. The disagreement about pain medication may look like a clinical disagreement. It may actually be the last round of an argument that started in 1987 about who loved the parent more. The medication is the vehicle. The argument is older.

Anticipatory loss of role is happening. When a parent dies, the adult children lose the roles they have held their whole lives as son or daughter of this person. Those roles were often how they knew themselves. Losing them is disorienting. The urgency to be the good daughter, or the one who did the right thing, or the one who was there, is partly about holding onto a version of the self that is about to change.

Guilt is in the room. Almost every adult child near a dying parent is carrying some guilt. Guilt about not visiting enough. Guilt about things said or not said. Guilt about earlier family decisions. The guilt does not usually present as guilt. It presents as anger at the sibling who seems to be making decisions that will increase the guilt.

Helplessness is driving behavior. The family cannot stop the disease. They cannot save the patient. The only decisions left are small ones about pain medication, about who visits when, about trying one more thing. Those small decisions carry the weight of all the large ones that nobody can make. People argue fiercely about small decisions when the large ones are impossible.

Understanding this does not make the conflict easier to manage. It does help you respond without taking sides. The sister who seems most combative is often the one carrying the most guilt. The brother who seems coldly rational is often the one trying hardest not to feel. The daughter who keeps bringing up things from the past is often the one who is not ready to lose her mother. None of them is wrong. All of them are working through something that looks like a disagreement about the patient but is actually a disagreement about themselves.

17.2 Reflecting Each Perspective

The MI move in a family disagreement is to reflect each perspective to the room, in the presence of the others. Not arguing. Not mediating. Reflecting.

When two family members are arguing, the instinct for most clinicians is to pick a side or to suggest a compromise. Neither works well. Picking a side turns the clinician into a third combatant. Suggesting a compromise often produces something nobody actually supports.

Reflecting each perspective, in front of the others, does something different. It names what each person is experiencing in a way that makes it visible to everyone in the room. Often the family members have never actually heard each other before. They have been reacting to what they assumed the other meant. When the clinician names what each person is really feeling, the others often hear it for the first time.

In the Oduya family, Amara could have said in the kitchen:

"Layla, you are terrified your father is suffering and you can't bear to watch him in pain. Gemma, you are terrified he is going to slip away before you have had the conversation you have been wanting to have with him. Both of you are telling me, in different ways, that you love him and you cannot stand what is happening to him."

Each sentence would be reflection of what Amara had heard. No compromise. No side. Just what each person is actually living with. Families who hear each other's real experience often stop fighting about the surface issue, because the surface issue is not the real issue.

The structure for reflecting to the room:

"Let me say back what I am hearing from each of you."

"[Name], what I hear from you is X, because Y matters to you."

"[Other name], what I hear from you is A, because B matters to you."

"Both of you are telling me something about how much you love [the patient]."

The last line is the move that often shifts the room. It names what is shared underneath the disagreement. Not "you both want him to be comfortable" (a claim about what they agree on, which may not be accurate). Not "you both love him" alone (too general to mean much). Something like "you are both telling me that what matters most is how he spends his last days, and you are seeing that differently." This names the shared concern without flattening the difference.

17.3 The Shared Value Underneath

Most family disagreements about end of life care, when examined carefully, rest on a shared value expressed differently. The siblings who disagree about morphine both want their father's last days to be good. They disagree about what "good" looks like. The siblings who disagree about hospice both want to care for their mother well. They disagree about what "well" means. The spouses who disagree about aggressive treatment both want to honor the patient. They disagree about how.

The facilitator's work is to find and name the shared value, without dismissing the disagreement about how to express it.

"You both want him to feel loved in his last days. You disagree about what that looks like."

"You both want to do right by her. You have different ideas about what doing right means."

"You both want to protect him from suffering. You disagree about what the biggest source of suffering is."

This framing does several things. It tells the family they are not actually enemies. It tells them the disagreement is about interpretation, not about values. It makes it easier to work the disagreement, because disagreement about interpretation can be negotiated. Disagreement about fundamental values usually cannot.

If you cannot find a shared value, keep looking. Often the shared value is deeper than the family realizes. They may both, at the root, want the patient to die with dignity. They may both want the other siblings to feel the care was done right. They may both want to feel they did enough. Going deeper often reveals a shared foundation even when the surface looks like conflict.

Occasionally there is no shared value. Sometimes a family member is genuinely motivated by something other than the patient's welfare. A son who wants to extend a dying parent's life for inheritance reasons. A daughter who wants to cut a sibling out of decisions for revenge. These situations exist. They are less common than they appear in the moment. When they do exist, the facilitator's job is to protect the patient, sometimes by centering the patient's expressed wishes and sometimes by involving an ethics committee or other external support.

But most of the time, the shared value is there. Finding it is the difference between a family meeting that fragments and a family meeting that holds.

17.4 A Real Example

Meet David. He was a palliative medicine physician at a large teaching hospital. His patient was a 79 year old man named Mr. Park with advanced heart failure. Mr. Park's three children were arguing about continuing his LVAD therapy.

The oldest son, Kenji, wanted to continue aggressive management. The middle daughter, Yuki, wanted to transition to comfort care. The youngest son, Akira, had been silent through most of the conversation until the argument escalated.

David did the rotation. Kenji talked about how his father had always been a fighter, how giving up on the LVAD was giving up on him. Yuki talked about how her father looked exhausted, how he had told her last month that he was tired. Akira said almost nothing.

David reflected Kenji: "You are worried that if we change what we are doing, it will feel to your father like we stopped fighting for him, and that is not what he would want."

Kenji said, "Yes."

David reflected Yuki: "You are worried that if we keep doing what we are doing, he will spend his last days with his body being pushed past what it can handle, and that is also not what he would want."

Yuki said, "Yes."

David then said something to both of them: "So both of you are trying to give him what he would want. The question is what he would want. You disagree about that. I want to ask Akira what he has been thinking. He has been quiet, and I want to make sure we hear him."

Akira said, "He told me last week he was tired. He also told me he did not want to disappoint any of you. I don't know what he would want if he did not have to worry about disappointing us."

The room went quiet. Yuki started to cry. Kenji sat back.

David said, "That is important information. Your father is trying not to disappoint you. That might be why none of us has heard from him clearly about what he wants. Is there a way the three of you could have a conversation with him, together, where you tell him that you support whatever he decides, and then listen to him?"

They did. Mr. Park told his three children together, for the first time, that he was ready to stop. Within a week, the LVAD was turned off. He died in his own bed, with all three of them present.

What this means for you: The shared value in the Park family was not agreement on what should happen medically. It was that all three children wanted to do right by their father. David's move was to frame their disagreement as two different versions of the same wish, and then to surface the fact that the father himself had not been clear because he was trying to protect them. The family's disagreement resolved when they stopped fighting each other and instead went to the father together.

17.5 When The Decision Maker Must Hold Firm

Not every family disagreement resolves through finding the shared value. Sometimes the legally designated decision maker has to make a call that some family members will not like. In those cases, the facilitator's job is not to produce consensus. It is to support the decision maker while the disagreement continues.

The healthcare proxy or durable power of attorney has legal authority to make decisions if the patient cannot. In many states, if there is no designated proxy, there is a hierarchy (spouse, adult child, etc.) that determines who decides. Whoever is in that role has the authority. They may or may not have the emotional bandwidth to hold firm against family pressure.

Your job, when the decision maker is being pressured by other family members to make a decision they do not believe is right, is to support the decision maker's authority without isolating the other family members.

Specific supports:

"Elena is the one your mother designated as the decision maker. She has been meeting with the medical team. She is making the decision based on what she knows about your mother's wishes. The rest of you have important roles too, but the final call is hers."

"I know you disagree. Elena has heard your disagreement. She is still going to make the call your mother asked her to make. We are going to honor that."

"It is your mother's wish that Elena be the one to decide. Respecting Elena's role is part of respecting your mother."

These supports do several things. They locate authority clearly. They connect the decision maker's role to the patient's expressed wishes, which is harder for the other family members to argue against. They leave the door open for the other family members to be involved in the care without being the deciders.

Sometimes the decision maker asks you to handle the other family members. "I can't deal with my brother. Can you talk to him?" This is a legitimate request. You can be the one who sits down with the dissenting family member, acknowledges their pain, reflects their concerns, and maintains the decision maker's authority. The separate conversation often reduces the pressure on the decision maker and gives the dissenter a chance to be heard by someone who is not emotionally entangled with them.

One note. If the decision maker is making a decision you believe is not in the patient's best interest (for example, pursuing aggressive treatment that the patient had clearly said they did not want), you have a different set of responsibilities. Those situations are complex and often involve ethics consultation. The focus of this chapter is the common situation where the decision maker is making a defensible decision and facing family resistance. In that situation, supporting them is usually the right move.

17.6 Another Real Example

Meet Fatima. She was a hospice social worker. Her patient was Mrs. Johnson, a 83 year old woman with dementia in hospice at a nursing facility. Her three children were her surrogate decision makers. Her oldest daughter, Aisha, had been taking the lead.

Mrs. Johnson had been declining for months. She had stopped eating a week ago. The question was continuing to offer food or transitioning to comfort feeding only. Aisha had reviewed the clinical information, talked with the team, and decided comfort feeding was what her mother would want.

Her brother, Marcus, disagreed. He flew in from Texas and immediately started talking to the staff about how his sister was "starving" their mother. The facility staff were stressed. Aisha was exhausted and starting to second guess herself.

Fatima met with Aisha alone first. She said, "I want to check in with you. You have made a decision that fits what you know about your mother. Your brother is pushing back. How are you doing with that?"

Aisha said, "I am starting to wonder if I am doing the right thing. Maybe he sees something I don't."

Fatima said, "Tell me what your mother told you she wanted, when she could still tell you."

Aisha said, "She told me she did not want to be kept alive by tubes or machines if she could not enjoy her life anymore. She said that at least a dozen times over the years."

Fatima said, "Has anything changed about what she told you?"

Aisha said, "No. But Marcus is making me doubt myself."

Fatima said, "Your mother did not put Marcus in charge. She put you in charge. Not because you are better than him, but because you were the one she had the conversations with. The decision is still yours, and it sounds like you have been making it based on what she told you."

Aisha started to cry. She said, "I know. I just hate that he is mad at me."

Fatima said, "That is real. Would it help if I talked with Marcus? I can acknowledge his pain without changing the decision."

Aisha said yes.

Fatima met with Marcus. She did not argue about the feeding. She asked him about his relationship with his mother. He talked for twenty minutes about being the youngest, about living far away, about not having been there for the last three years. He cried.

Fatima said, "You are mad because you feel like you are losing her and you have not had the time you wanted with her."

Marcus said, "Yes."

Fatima said, "I want to tell you something that I do not think Aisha has been able to say to you. Your sister is not starving your mother. Your sister is honoring what your mother asked her to honor. She is doing it alone, while also trying to protect you. The anger you are feeling at her is real, but it is not about the feeding. It is about something else."

Marcus was quiet for a long time. He said, "I don't know what to do with this."

Fatima said, "Go sit with your mother. Tell her what you have not said. She may not hear the words, but say them anyway. That is the thing you can still do."

He did. Mrs. Johnson died three days later. Marcus and Aisha spoke at the funeral. They have not fully reconciled. They have not fought again.

What this means for you: Supporting the decision maker does not mean shutting down the dissenter. The decision maker needs someone to reaffirm their authority. The dissenter needs someone to acknowledge their pain and redirect their energy. Both roles can be played by the same facilitator, in separate conversations, without compromising either. The decision holds because the authority is clear. The relationship has a chance to heal because the dissenter was met with care.

17.7 Boundaries On Conflict In Front Of The Patient

One thing that does not get negotiated is open conflict in front of a patient who is dying.

A patient who can hear should not have to listen to family members fighting about their care. A patient who cannot clearly hear is often more aware than family members realize. Dying patients often report, in the rare cases where they later recover, having heard conversations that took place around their beds when everyone assumed they were not aware.

Setting this as a bright line is part of the facilitator's job.

"I am going to interrupt. This conversation cannot happen in this room. We are going to continue it somewhere else."

"Your father can hear you. Whatever disagreement you have, take it outside."

"I need everyone to stop. We are going to finish this in the hallway. Your mother does not need to hear this."

These lines are delivered without apology and without anger. They are a boundary, not a critique. Most family members, when redirected, take the cue immediately. They have been caught up in the emotion and have lost track of where they are. Naming it brings them back.

Sometimes a family member will push back. "She can't hear us. She's been out of it for days." The response is firm. "She may or may not be able to hear. We are not going to take that chance. This conversation happens outside."

There are two reasons for this bright line. The first is the patient's dignity. The second, and often underappreciated, is the family members' own long term wellbeing. A son who spent his father's last hour fighting with his sister in front of him will carry that memory for decades. Preventing the memory from being created is protective for him, not just for the patient.

Once the family is outside, the facilitator can work with the conflict. Reflections. Shared values. Decision maker support. All the tools in this chapter. The work happens. Just not at the bedside.

When the family comes back into the room, help them transition. "Before we go back in, let's take a breath. Whatever you are going to say in there, it is going to be for your father. Not for each other." This moment of transition helps them walk in as caregivers rather than as combatants.

17.8 When It Does Not Work

The most common failure in managing family disagreement is that the facilitator tries to resolve the disagreement when the disagreement is not actually about what it looks like. The clinician mediates the argument about the medication. A day later, there is a new argument about the nursing shift. A day after that, an argument about the hospice chaplain. The surface topic keeps changing. The underlying dynamic does not.

Three things to try:

1. When a family keeps generating new disagreements, suspect that the disagreements are not the point. The point is some underlying dynamic, usually old, that is expressing itself through whatever topic is available. Mediating the surface topics will not help. Naming the underlying dynamic, with care, sometimes does. 2. If you cannot name the dynamic, try asking a family member privately. "I notice your family keeps finding things to disagree about. Do you have a sense of what is really going on?" Often one family member knows. They have been waiting for someone to ask. 3. When the dynamic is too old or too deep for anyone to name it in the current moment, shift your role. Stop trying to produce family harmony. Start trying to ensure the patient is protected and the necessary decisions get made. Some families will not heal before the patient dies. Your job is not to force them. Your job is to ensure the dying is as good as it can be given what the family brought into the room.

A second failure is taking sides. A clinician who has come to believe one family member is right and the others are wrong often stops being effective. They start subtly advocating for the one they agree with. The others feel it. The meeting fragments. If you find yourself siding, step back. Bring in a colleague. Be honest with yourself about why you are taking the side you are. Sometimes the feeling is rooted in genuine clinical judgment. Sometimes it is rooted in something personal that the family situation is activating in you. Either way, the taking of sides compromises your ability to facilitate.

17.9 What To Take Away

Family disagreement near the end of life is not primarily about the topic the family is arguing about. It is about grief arriving differently in different people, unfinished business surfacing, guilt, helplessness, and the anticipated loss of roles that family members have held their whole lives. Understanding the mechanism lets you respond to the real thing rather than the surface disagreement.

The MI move is to reflect each perspective to the room. Not to mediate. Not to compromise. To name what each person is experiencing, in front of the others, so they hear each other for possibly the first time. The move often shifts the room, because what looks like two opposing positions is often two different expressions of the same underlying concern.

Locating the shared value underneath the dispute is the work that lets families find their way. "You both want him to be at peace, and you are seeing different paths to that" is a different frame from "you disagree about the medication." The first frame is solvable. The second often is not.

Sometimes the decision maker has to hold firm despite family disagreement. Your job is to support them clearly, to acknowledge the other family members without redirecting authority, and sometimes to handle the dissenters in separate conversations so the decision maker can focus on the patient.

Open conflict in front of a dying patient is one of the few things that does not get negotiated. Set the boundary firmly and kindly. Move the conflict to the hallway. Work it there. Bring everyone back into the room as caregivers, not as combatants.

The next chapter handles a specific form of family disagreement that comes up often enough to deserve its own treatment. The absent relative who arrives late, who has not been part of the decision making, and who arrives with intensity that destabilizes the plan the family has already made. Chapter 18.0 is about working with them without letting their arrival undo what came before.

Chapter 18: The Absent Relative Who Arrives

Mrs. Patel had been in a skilled nursing facility for three months on hospice for end stage heart failure. Her husband and her daughter Gemma, who lived in the same city, had been at her bedside almost daily. The hospice team knew them well. The care plan had been built over weeks of conversations. Mrs. Patel was comfortable. She was sleeping most of the time. She was expected to die within days to weeks.

On a Monday morning, Gemma's brother Raj arrived from Seattle. He had not been home in two years. He had not been involved in any of the medical decisions. He had called weekly, but the calls had been brief.

He walked into his mother's room, stayed for fifteen minutes, and came out demanding a family meeting. In the meeting, he said he wanted his mother transferred to a major academic medical center for "a second opinion." He wanted to know why she was not on IV fluids. He wanted to know why she was not getting more aggressive treatment. He was angry. He accused his sister of "letting their mother die without fighting."

Gemma started crying. The father sat silent, torn between his two children. The hospice medical director, a woman named Aisha, watched Raj escalate for about three minutes. Then she said something that changed the meeting.

She said, "Raj, I can see this is very hard for you. You have come a long way and your mother is dying. Before we talk about any medical decisions, I want to ask you something. When did you last speak with your mother, really speak, when she was still clear?"

Raj said, "Six months ago. On her birthday."

Aisha said, "What did she say to you then, about what she wanted?"

Raj was quiet for a long time. He said, "She told me she was tired. She said she did not want to go back to the hospital again. She said she wanted to die at home, or somewhere like home."

The room went quiet.

Aisha said, "What your sister and father have been doing is honoring what your mother told you six months ago. She told you what she wanted. They are following it."

Raj started to cry. He sat down. He said, "I didn't know what else to do. I walked in and she looked so small. I thought I had to do something."

Aisha said, "You can still do something. You can be here. You can sit with her. You can hold her hand. That is the thing she needed from you, not a transfer."

The meeting ended without a transfer order. Raj stayed for four days. His mother died on the third day, with her husband, her daughter, and her son at her bedside.

This chapter is about that specific pattern. The absent relative who arrives at the end and tries to change the plan. You will learn why late arrivers escalate, what the guilt and grief under the demand usually are, how to reflect without siding with anyone, how to reorient the conversation toward the patient's own voice, and how to protect the primary caregiver from the destabilization that a late arriver can bring.

18.1 Why Late Arrivers Escalate

The pattern is consistent enough across families that it is worth naming. A relative who has been absent from the caregiving arrives, often shortly before the end. Within hours or days of arrival, they become the most intense voice in the room. They question decisions that have been carefully made. They demand more aggressive intervention, or sometimes less, depending on what they find. They generate conflict where there had been relative calm.

This is not about bad character. It is about what the situation is doing to them.

Guilt is the driver. The late arriver knows, consciously or not, that they have not been present in the way the other family members have. They are walking into a room where a sibling has been at the bedside for months. They are meeting nursing staff who know their parent's preferences better than they do. They feel, immediately, the gap between what they have done and what others have done. The feeling is unbearable. It expresses as something else.

Shock plays a role. The late arriver has been hearing about the decline by phone. Phone calls compress and soften information. The reality, seen in person, is worse than any phone call prepared them for. The parent they remember from a year ago is not the parent in the bed. The gap between expectation and reality produces a kind of shock that the primary caregivers have been absorbing slowly over months. The late arriver absorbs it in fifteen minutes. The response is often to insist that something has gone wrong. Somebody must have made mistakes. Otherwise the parent would not look this bad.

Lost time is being mourned. The late arriver knows, in the moment of arrival, that they will not have the time they wanted. There will not be the long conversation. There will not be the reconciliation they had imagined. There will not be the chance to make up for the distance. The grief about this is already present before the death. It is disguised as insistence on fixing something that cannot be fixed.

Being useful is a last ditch attempt at meaning. The late arriver cannot rewind their absence. They can try to do something now. Demanding a transfer, demanding a new treatment, demanding a second opinion. These are attempts to contribute something tangible to a situation they have not contributed to. The demands are often impractical or counterproductive, but the impulse behind them is an attempt to matter.

Understanding these dynamics is the foundation for working with them. The late arriver is not a villain. They are a person drowning in what they have not done, trying to do something now that proves they still love the parent. Meeting them with judgment amplifies the drowning. Meeting them with compassion, while also holding the existing plan, is the move.

18.2 Guilt And Grief Under The Demand

Most demands from late arrivers are expressions of guilt and grief, not of careful medical opinions. If you respond to the demand at face value, you will miss what is actually happening.

The demand: "I want her transferred to University Hospital for a second opinion." Underneath: "I feel terrible that I was not here, and I need to believe something more could be done, because if everything possible has already been done, then the guilt is final."

The demand: "Why is she not on a feeding tube?" Underneath: "I cannot watch my mother starve, and I need to fix something, because sitting here doing nothing is impossible to bear."

The demand: "Who decided this?" Underneath: "I was not part of this decision and I need to understand how it was made without me, because being excluded feels like being told I do not count."

Responding to the surface demand usually fails. You explain why transfer is not medically indicated. The late arriver argues with the explanation. You explain again. The argument escalates. By the end, neither of you has touched what is actually driving the demand.

The move is to acknowledge the underneath, carefully.

"Raj, I hear you asking about transfer, and I want to talk about that. Before we do, I want to name something. You just arrived. You have not had time to absorb what has been happening. You are seeing your mother in a state that is very different from when you last saw her. That is a lot. Can we talk about what you are walking into before we talk about what to do next?"

"I am hearing you say you want the feeding tube. Before we talk about feeding, can I ask what you are holding right now? You came a long way. You are seeing her in a condition you were not prepared for. What is it like for you?"

"I know you were not part of the earlier meetings. I want to walk you through what has been decided, and why, and then we can talk about any questions you have about it. You deserve to understand how we got here."

Each of these moves slows the conversation down. It addresses the human first and the demand second. When the late arriver is actually met, the demand often softens or disappears. It was not really about the surface thing. It was about needing to be seen in their particular grief.

18.3 Reflecting Without Siding

When a late arriver arrives and starts making demands, the primary caregivers often feel attacked. They have been doing the work. They know the patient's wishes. They resent the implication that they have been doing it wrong. The instinct of the facilitator is to defend them. This instinct is wrong.

Defending the primary caregivers in front of the late arriver does two bad things. It puts the late arriver in opposition to the clinician, which makes the conversation combative rather than therapeutic. It also denies the late arriver the acknowledgment of their own pain, which is the thing they need most.

The move is to reflect the late arriver without siding against the primary caregivers. You hear them. You name what they are experiencing. You do not confirm that their demand is correct. You also do not deny it. You hold the frame that everyone in the room is in pain, including them.

"Raj, you got here last night. You walked in and saw your mother in a way that was very hard. You are now in a meeting where other people have been making decisions for months without you. That is a lot. I want you to know I see that."

No agreement with the demand. No defense of the caregivers. Just acknowledgment of his experience.

Then you can broaden the frame to include everyone.

"I also want to acknowledge that your father and your sister have been here. They have been making hard decisions under hard conditions. They have been trying to honor what your mother wanted. You are all in pain. Your pain looks different from their pain, because you have come into this at a different moment. But all of you are in pain."

This framing does not resolve anything. It does name that everyone is struggling. It prevents the conversation from becoming Raj versus Gemma. It prepares the room for the real work of reorienting to the patient's voice.

Sometimes the late arriver will push back against this framing. "My sister has not been making hard decisions, she has been giving up." At this point, do not argue. Reflect. "You are worried that what has been happening has been giving up rather than honoring your mother." Wait. "Can I share what I have seen?" If they say yes, you can describe, briefly, what you have observed of the primary caregivers' work, without making it into a defense.

The frame you want to hold is: everyone loves her, everyone is in pain, everyone is doing what they can with what they have. When that frame is in the room, the conflict often deflates. When the frame is missing, the conflict often escalates.

18.4 Reorienting To The Patient

Once the late arriver has been met, the move is to reorient the conversation toward the patient's own voice.

The late arriver has been operating in a register of "what should be done about her." That register is about the family's action. The reorienting move is to shift to "what has she said she wants."

"I want to ask you, Raj, a different question. You talked to your mother on her birthday six months ago. Before that, you have known her your whole life. What did she tell you, over the years, about how she wanted her last days to go?"

"What do you know about your mother's wishes? Not what the doctors have decided. Not what your sister thinks. What did your mother tell you?"

"If your mother could speak to us right now, what do you think she would say about what is happening?"

These questions change the subject. They move from "what are we going to do" to "what did she want." They also activate something in the late arriver that often cannot be activated in the middle of a demand. Most late arrivers, when asked this question sincerely, know something about what their parent wanted. They may have been avoiding that knowledge, because acknowledging it makes the current plan harder to fight.

When the late arriver accesses their own memory of what the parent wanted, the demand often shifts on its own. They hear themselves say that their mother did not want to be in a hospital. They hear themselves say that their father hated tubes. They hear themselves say that their parent had been ready to stop fighting for months. Once they hear themselves say these things, the demand for aggressive intervention is harder to sustain.

You do not have to argue with the demand. The late arriver's own memory of the parent, surfaced carefully, often does the argument for you.

18.5 A Real Example

Meet Elena. She was a hospice social worker in her eighth year. Her patient was Mr. Thompson, an 86 year old man with advanced dementia in the late stages. He had been at home on hospice for six weeks. His wife Fatima had been the primary caregiver. Their daughter, who lived nearby, had been a supporting caregiver.

Their son Omar arrived from Chicago on a Friday evening. He had not visited in nine months. He walked into the bedroom, saw his father unresponsive and breathing with a rattle, and walked out angry. He told Fatima he wanted his father admitted to the hospital. He was furious that his father was dying at home.

Elena came out on Saturday morning. She asked Fatima to give her twenty minutes with Omar.

She sat on the porch with Omar. She did not explain anything. She said, "You got in last night. What was it like walking in?"

Omar said, "He didn't look like my dad."

Elena said, "He is not the man you remember."

Omar said, "No. And my sister has been letting this happen. And my mom is exhausted and doesn't seem to know what day it is. And nobody called me. Nobody told me it was this bad."

Elena said, "You are angry that nobody told you how bad it was, and you are also angry at yourself for not knowing."

Omar was quiet. He said, "I should have come home a long time ago."

Elena said, "Yes."

She did not soften that yes. She let it sit.

Then she said, "You are here now. What would your father want you to do now, given that you are here and he is dying."

Omar said, "I don't know."

Elena said, "What did he tell you, when he could still tell you?"

Omar thought for a while. He said, "He told me he never wanted to be kept alive on machines. He told me, many times, that if he got dementia, he did not want anyone doing anything to prolong it. He said it was the worst thing he could imagine."

Elena said, "So what your family has been doing is honoring what he asked for."

Omar said, "Yes."

Elena said, "What do you want to do now, with what you have."

Omar said, "I want to sit with him."

He went inside. He sat with his father for the rest of Saturday. He did not demand a transfer again. His father died on Sunday afternoon, with Omar and Fatima at the bedside. The daughter arrived ten minutes after the death.

Omar cried for an hour. Then he said to Elena, "Thank you for not letting me do the thing I was going to do."

What this means for you: Sometimes the most helpful move with a late arriver is to let their own guilt be named, without rescuing them from it. Elena did not reassure Omar that he was not at fault. She let him see that he had missed time, and then she gave him a way to use what he had left. The demand for a transfer was really a way of not sitting with his father. Once Omar was able to sit, the demand was no longer necessary.

18.6 Another Real Example

Meet Marcus. He was a palliative medicine physician on an inpatient team. His patient was Mrs. Ofori, a 79 year old woman with metastatic breast cancer. She was expected to die within days. Her husband, three of her four children, and several grandchildren had been present for weeks. The fourth child, Kenji, had been estranged from the family for eight years after a financial dispute.

Kenji arrived on a Wednesday afternoon. He went into his mother's room, spoke with her briefly, came out, and demanded a family meeting. He was not angry about the medical care. He was angry about being excluded from the estate conversation that had happened two months ago. He wanted to litigate that in the meeting.

Marcus saw what was happening. He convened the meeting. Kenji started to talk about the estate.

Marcus said, "Kenji, I am going to stop you. I want to say something clearly. The estate conversation is not going to happen in this room. That is a conversation for another time, with another facilitator, possibly with lawyers. I am not the right person to help with that, and your mother's final days are not the right time or place."

Kenji started to argue. Marcus continued.

"You are here. Your mother is dying. What I can help with is how you want to spend the time you have left with her. I cannot help with eight years of what happened between you and your siblings. That is not in my scope, and it is not fair to your mother's dying to put it in this room."

Kenji sat back. He said, "So what am I supposed to do."

Marcus said, "You are supposed to sit with your mother if you want to. You are supposed to tell her what you want her to know. You can do that alone, or with your father. The rest of it can wait."

Kenji was quiet for a long time. He said, "What if I do not want to see her without dealing with the estate stuff first?"

Marcus said, "Then you do not see her. That is your choice. But you do not get to make the last days of her life be about the estate. That part is a line I am going to hold."

Kenji went to the hospital cafeteria. He came back two hours later. He sat with his mother for the rest of the evening. He did not bring up the estate again. She died the next morning.

What this means for you: Sometimes a late arriver is bringing something into the room that does not belong in the room. Family conflicts that predate the dying do not have to be worked out at the bedside. Naming the line, firmly and kindly, is part of the facilitator's role. The patient's dying is not the right container for every family wound. You can acknowledge the wound, decline to address it in the current setting, and redirect the late arriver to what is possible.

18.7 Protecting The Primary Caregiver

The arrival of a late relative is often hardest on the primary caregiver. They have been doing the work. They have been making decisions. They have been exhausted. Now a sibling or spouse arrives and questions their decisions and their care.

Your job is to protect the primary caregiver's autonomy and their role, while also not excluding the late arriver.

Specific protections:

Do not let the late arriver override a decision that has been carefully made. If the late arriver is trying to reverse a plan the family has agreed to and the patient has endorsed, support the existing plan. "The plan that is in place was made after a lot of thought. It was made with what your mother told us she wanted. We are not reopening it."

Do not let the late arriver criticize the primary caregiver's work. When a late arriver starts to criticize, acknowledge their feelings but redirect. "You are frustrated that you were not part of earlier decisions. That is real. It is not fair to turn that frustration into criticism of your sister, who has been here doing the work." This sentence supports the caregiver without shaming the late arriver.

Do not let the primary caregiver have to defend themselves alone. If a late arriver is questioning the caregiver in front of the whole family, step in. "Let me answer some of what you are asking about the plan. These are medical decisions, and I am the right person to explain them." This takes the burden off the caregiver and puts the answering in the hands of someone with clinical authority.

Consider separate conversations. The late arriver often benefits from a one on one conversation with the facilitator, away from the primary caregiver. This lets the late arriver express what they are holding without attacking the caregiver. It also gives the caregiver a break from the emotional work of managing the new arrival.

Check on the primary caregiver after. The primary caregiver has usually been bracing for the arrival. Once the arriver is there, the caregiver often crashes. Find them. Acknowledge what they are carrying. "This is a lot on top of what you were already carrying. How are you doing?" The caregiver may not have been asked that in weeks.

One last protection. If the late arriver is persistently disruptive, it is appropriate to limit their access to the patient or to family decisions. This is rare. When it is needed, it is usually a decision made with the primary caregiver and the patient's healthcare proxy, not unilaterally by the clinician. Most late arrivers, met with compassion, do not require this level of intervention. But the option exists, and in the rare situations where it is needed, your willingness to name it protects the patient and the primary caregiver from continued harm.

18.8 When It Does Not Work

The most common failure with late arrivers is that the facilitator tries to produce reconciliation between the late arriver and the primary caregiver during the patient's dying. This is rarely possible. The time is wrong. The stakes are too high. The emotional bandwidth is spent.

Three things to try:

1. Lower the goal. The goal during the dying is not reconciliation. It is containment. The goal is that the late arriver does not destabilize the existing plan, and that the primary caregiver is not consumed by managing the arriver. Reconciliation, if it happens, will happen over months or years after the death, not in the last few days. 2. Redirect energy. If the late arriver has energy to burn, find something for them to do that does not involve decision making. Some late arrivers are helpful with coordinating visitors, with running errands, with sitting with the patient overnight so the primary caregiver can sleep. Giving them a role other than decision maker channels the guilt driven energy into something useful. 3. Set clear containers. "You can be here. You can sit with her. You can participate in certain conversations. You are not in charge of the medical decisions, because the healthcare proxy is. I am not asking you to agree with everything. I am asking you to not disrupt what is already in place." This kind of clear containment is often a relief rather than a restriction. Late arrivers are sometimes looking for someone to tell them what the limits are.

A second failure is being too hard on the late arriver. The guilt the late arriver is carrying is often crushing. If the facilitator piles on judgment, even subtly, the late arriver will either double down on their demands or collapse into shame that makes them less present with the patient. Compassion for the late arriver is not indulgence. It is the practical thing that makes the dying go better for everyone.

18.9 The Quick Version

The late arriver pattern is common enough to be predictable. A relative who has been absent arrives near the end. Within hours or days, they are the most intense voice in the room. They demand changes to the plan. They question decisions. They generate conflict.

The driver is almost always guilt, grief, shock, and a last ditch attempt at meaning, rather than bad character. The demand for a transfer is usually not about medical judgment. It is about needing to do something, to prove they still love the parent, to fix what has been left undone.

Responding to the surface demand usually fails. The move is to meet the underneath. Slow the conversation down. Acknowledge what they are walking into. Ask what they know about what the patient wanted. Reflect their pain without siding against the primary caregivers.

Reorient to the patient's voice. Most late arrivers, when asked what the parent told them over the years, know something real. Surfacing that knowledge often shifts the demand without argument.

Protect the primary caregiver. Do not let the late arriver override decisions that have been carefully made. Step in when criticism starts. Offer the late arriver a role that is not decision making. Check on the caregiver after the late arriver's visit.

Lower the goal. The dying is not the time for family reconciliation. Containment is enough. Reconciliation, if it happens, will happen later. What matters now is that the patient's final days reflect the patient's own wishes, that the primary caregiver is supported, and that the late arriver is met with enough compassion to not destabilize what came before.

With Part IV complete, the book turns to specific populations and contexts in Part V. Dementia and the lost voice, pediatric palliative care, cultural considerations. The skills you have built across the first four parts all apply. The next three chapters adapt them for situations that require specific care.

18.10 Reference List

Byock, I. (2004). The four things that matter most: A book about living. Atria Books.

Chambers Evans, J., and Carnevale, F. A. (2005). Dawning of awareness: The experience of surrogate decision making at the end of life. Journal of Clinical Ethics, 16(1), 28 45. https://pubmed.ncbi.nlm.nih.gov/16032980/

Kramer, B. J., and Yonker, J. A. (2011). Perceived success in addressing end of life care needs of low income elders and their families: What has family conflict got to do with it? Journal of Pain and Symptom Management, 41(1), 35 48. https://doi.org/10.1016/j.jpainsymman.2010.04.017

Norris, W. M., Nielsen, E. L., Engelberg, R. A., and Curtis, J. R. (2005). Treatment preferences for resuscitation and critical care among homeless persons. Chest, 127(6), 2180 2187. https://doi.org/10.1378/chest.127.6.2180

Radwany, S., Albanese, T., Clough, L., Sims, L., Mason, H., and Jahangiri, S. (2009). End of life decision making and emotional burden: Placing family meetings in context. American Journal of Hospice and Palliative Medicine, 26(5), 376 383. https://doi.org/10.1177/1049909109338515

Rolland, J. S. (1994). Families, illness, and disability: An integrative treatment model. Basic Books.

Teno, J. M., Clarridge, B. R., Casey, V., Welch, L. C., Wetle, T., Shield, R., and Mor, V. (2004). Family perspectives on end of life care at the last place of care. JAMA, 291(1), 88 93. https://doi.org/10.1001/jama.291.1.88

Van Scoy, L. J., Reading, J. M., Scott, A. M., Chuang, C., and Levi, B. H. (2016). Conversation Game effectively engages groups of individuals in discussions about death and dying. Journal of Palliative Medicine, 19(6), 661 667. https://doi.org/10.1089/jpm.2015.0390

Washington, K. T., Demiris, G., Parker Oliver, D., Swarz, J., and Lewis, A. M. (2012). Delivering problem solving therapy to family caregivers of people with cancer: A feasibility study in outpatient palliative care. Psycho Oncology, 21(10), 1060 1066. https://doi.org/10.1002/pon.1995

Williams, A. L., and McCorkle, R. (2011). Cancer family caregivers during the palliative, hospice, and bereavement phases: A review of the descriptive psychosocial literature. Palliative and Supportive Care, 9(3), 315 325. https://doi.org/10.1017/S1478951511000265

PART V: SPECIAL POPULATIONS AND CONTEXTS

Chapter 19: Dementia And The Lost Voice

Mrs. Abara had written the advance directive in 2014. It was three pages. It was specific. She had wanted no ventilator support if she were in an irreversible condition. She had wanted no feeding tube if she could no longer recognize her family. She had wanted "to die with dignity," a phrase she had underlined.

It was now 2026. She was 84. She had been in a memory care unit for three years with advanced Alzheimer's disease. She no longer recognized her daughter most days. She did not speak in full sentences. She did not know her own name when asked.

And every morning, at about 7:30, she hummed. The same four notes. She smiled while she did it. The nursing aide, a woman named Ananya, had figured out it was the opening phrase of "Bring Him Home" from Les Misérables. Mrs. Abara had sung it in a community choir for twenty years. Ananya put it on a small speaker one morning. Mrs. Abara's face changed. She reached out her hand, trembling, and swayed in her wheelchair, her eyes closed.

On a Tuesday in February, Mrs. Abara developed a urinary tract infection. It became septic. She was admitted to the hospital. The internist wanted to know, from Mrs. Abara's daughter, about transferring her to the ICU if her blood pressure dropped further. The advance directive, written in 2014, said no aggressive intervention if she was in an irreversible condition. The daughter, Gemma, held the document in one hand and her mother's hand in the other. She looked up at the nurse practitioner, a woman named Amara, who had been brought in from palliative care.

Gemma said, "I know what the paper says. I don't know if the paper is still her."

This chapter is about the work that starts in that sentence. You will meet the distinction between substituted judgment and best interest standards, learn how to elicit the patient's voice through the family's memory, practice reading non verbal cues as real communication, face the hard question of what to do when past values and present expressions disagree, and learn how to use the FAST scale as a tool for hospice conversations with families.

19.1 Substituted Judgment And Best Interest

When a patient has lost capacity, clinicians rely on two different legal and ethical standards for making decisions.

Substituted judgment asks: what would this person have wanted, given what we know about their values, their history, and their previously expressed wishes? It places the patient's own voice, as remembered through their former self, at the center of the decision.

Best interest asks: what is most likely to promote this person's wellbeing right now, given their current state and circumstances? It places the patient's present welfare at the center, without necessarily referring to what they would have wanted.

These standards often produce the same answer. Mrs. Abara did not want to die in an ICU. Her current state, with sepsis, likely makes an ICU transfer more painful than beneficial. Substituted judgment and best interest both point toward not transferring.

Sometimes they diverge. A patient who, in a prior document, refused all feeding tubes now happily accepts spoon feeding. A patient who said they never wanted to live in a nursing home is now settled, apparently content, in one. A patient who signed a DNR years ago is now laughing at jokes with her grandchildren and looks, by any present measure, like someone who wants to stay alive. The past self said one thing. The present self is saying something different, through their body and their behavior.

Neither standard is always right. The legal default in most jurisdictions is substituted judgment when known, with best interest as the fallback. But in practice, the experienced clinician holds both. The patient's past wishes are one source of data. The patient's present responses are another. Both deserve weight.

The discipline is to ask both questions in every conversation.

What did this person say they wanted?

What does this person seem to want now?

If the answers match, the decision is clearer. If they differ, the family and the clinical team have real work to do, and the rest of this chapter is about how to do it.

19.2 Voice Through Memory

For patients who can no longer speak for themselves, the family's memory is often the richest source of information about who they are. This is not about pulling out a signed document. It is about eliciting stories, patterns, and examples that reveal what the patient has oriented around their entire life.

The elicitation uses the same open question skills from Part II, applied to the family rather than to the patient.

"Tell me about your mother before she got sick."

"What did she care about most?"

"What did a good day look like for her, ten years ago?"

"What kinds of things made her angry? What made her happy?"

"If she could see herself right now, what would she say?"

"What did she say to you, over the years, about how she wanted things to go if she got seriously sick?"

Listen. Reflect. Ask more. Let the family build the picture. By the time you are done, you have a much richer sense of who the patient is than any advance directive can contain.

This matters because advance directives, no matter how well written, almost never anticipate the specific situation the patient ends up in. The directive says "no feeding tube if I am not able to recognize my family." The current reality is that she does not recognize her daughter most days but lights up when her daughter sings to her. Does the directive apply? Does her response to the singing count as recognition? A document cannot answer that. A family who has been asked about who she is can help.

One specific move to recommend to families, if they ask: keep a journal of the patient's responses. Over a week, note when she smiled, what she ate willingly, what seemed to cause her distress. This is data. Clinicians who walk into a room cold do not see patterns. Families who have been paying attention often do. The patterns are what tell you what the patient is currently experiencing, which is crucial for decisions under either substituted judgment or best interest.

Another move. Ask about specific past comments. Most patients, before they lost capacity, said something about what they did or did not want. These comments are often remembered by family members but rarely surface in formal conversations. "Your mother ever said anything, offhand, about people she knew who had dementia? About how she'd feel about being in a place like this?" Those offhand comments are often closer to the patient's real values than the formal advance directive.

19.3 Reading Non Verbal Cues

A patient who can no longer speak in sentences is still communicating. The communication is in the body. Posture. Facial expression. Vocalizations. Response to touch, music, food, familiar voices. Reading these cues as real communication is a skill that many clinicians never develop, partly because medical training privileges verbal report over everything else.

Concrete cues to watch for:

Facial expression during care. A patient who grimaces when a certain caregiver approaches is communicating something. A patient who smiles when a specific voice comes on the phone is communicating something else.

Responses to specific stimuli. Music is a particularly powerful cue. Many patients with advanced dementia retain strong musical memory long after language is gone. A patient's response to their own favorite music, compared to unfamiliar music, can tell you a lot about what they are still experiencing.

Feeding behavior. A patient who turns her head away from certain foods and opens her mouth for others is telling you something. A patient who spits out liquid is telling you something. Feeding is communication, and it is often clearer than anything verbal.

Vocalizations. Groans. Rhythmic sounds. Word fragments. Crying. Laughter. The specific vocalization, and the context in which it occurs, carries information.

Body positioning. Does the patient curl toward a visitor or pull away? Does she relax her body when a familiar hand is on hers, or tense up?

These cues are data. They are admissible evidence in the clinical conversation. A family who says "she seems miserable" has information you should weigh. A family who says "she seems at peace" has information you should weigh. Neither is a decisive answer. Both are relevant.

The research on non verbal communication in dementia care supports this approach. Patients with advanced dementia retain emotional responsiveness long after cognitive function has largely declined (Kolanowski et al., 2011). Clinicians who learn to read non verbal cues report that patients who were thought to be "unreachable" are often responsive, just in ways that require different attention.

One clinical tool that helps is systematic pain assessment for patients who cannot self report. The PAINAD scale (Pain Assessment in Advanced Dementia) assigns scores based on breathing, vocalization, facial expression, body language, and consolability (Warden et al., 2003). Tools like this formalize what a skilled observer would already be doing. They are useful not because they produce a number, but because they discipline the observation.

19.4 When Past And Present Disagree

The hardest decisions in dementia care come when the past self and the present self are not in agreement.

A woman in her 60s wrote a directive saying she wanted no food or water if she could not recognize her children. She is now in her 80s, in late stage dementia, and eats with apparent pleasure when her aide feeds her small bites of applesauce.

A man said, years ago, that he would rather die than live in a nursing home. He has been living in a memory care unit for two years. He smiles when the staff come in. He holds hands. He is not the person he used to be, but he is not unhappy.

A woman signed a DNR in 2019, saying she would not want to be resuscitated. She is now having a cardiac event. She is conscious, looking at the nurse, and clearly frightened.

In each of these cases, the past directive and the present experience diverge. What do you do.

There is no universal answer. There are better and worse ways to work the question.

First, do not assume the past wins automatically. The past self was making decisions about a future self that did not yet exist. That future self is now here, with different experiences and, by all apparent measures, different responses. To ignore her is to privilege a theoretical person over a real one.

Second, do not assume the present wins automatically. The present self is often not in a position to hold a consistent set of values. Dementia can produce moment to moment preferences that do not reflect any stable wish. The woman who eats applesauce today might not eat tomorrow. Privileging the present moment without context can produce care that has no coherent direction.

Third, look for whichever signal is stronger and more stable. If the patient's present responses are consistent over weeks and appear to reflect a settled state, they deserve weight. If the present responses are inconsistent, reactive, or driven by confusion, they deserve less weight. If the past directive was written carefully, after reflection, in the context of similar situations, it deserves more weight. If the past directive was written in the abstract and does not quite fit the current circumstances, it deserves less.

Fourth, bring the family into the weighing. They knew the patient before. They are the ones who can tell you if her present responses look like her, or if they are something new that she would not have recognized.

An honest clinician conversation with the family sounds something like this.

"Your mother wrote this directive twelve years ago. It said she did not want a feeding tube if she could not recognize family. Right now, she is not recognizing most of you, and she is also eating with what looks like pleasure when we feed her by hand. I want to think about this with you. The old directive is one thing. The current experience is another. I don't want to mechanically apply the directive if it doesn't fit what is actually happening. I also don't want to override her stated wishes without thinking carefully. What do you think?"

This conversation honors both sources of information. It puts the family in the position of helping to weigh, rather than being handed a decision. It also acknowledges that the clinician does not have a clean answer. That honesty usually produces better decisions than pretending the directive alone answers the question.

19.5 A Real Example

Meet Marcus. He was a hospice medical director in his seventh year. His patient was Mr. Oduya, an 82 year old man with advanced vascular dementia. Mr. Oduya had written a directive years earlier: no artificial nutrition, no hospitalization, no aggressive treatment.

Mr. Oduya had aspirated twice in the last month. The long term care facility wanted to transfer him to the hospital for evaluation. Marcus met with the family. The family was tense. Mr. Oduya's son, Kwame, said he thought his father would want to be in the hospital "just to be checked." His daughter, Yuki, said the directive was clear and they should not transfer.

Marcus did not arbitrate. He said, "Tell me about your father before all this."

Kwame and Yuki talked for twenty five minutes. They told stories. They laughed a few times. Their father had been a retired mechanical engineer. He had built his own house. He had refused to use contractors because "he knew what he wanted better than any stranger." He had taken the bus to doctor's appointments even in his seventies because "hospitals are where people go to lose themselves." He had visited his own mother in a nursing home for eight years and had said afterward, "I am never going there. Never."

Marcus reflected: "Your father's whole life was about doing things his own way, in his own home, on his own terms. He did not trust hospitals. He had watched his own mother disappear in one."

Kwame sat quietly.

Marcus said, "It sounds like the hospital trip is not what your father would want."

Kwame said, "I know. I was just scared."

Yuki took her brother's hand.

Marcus said, "Being scared is normal. It does not mean you have to do something he would not have wanted."

They decided against the transfer. Mr. Oduya was managed at the facility with comfort measures. He died eleven days later, in the bed he had been in for the last two years, with both children at his side.

What this means for you: Substituted judgment becomes real when the family tells stories about who the person was. The stories carry the values. The values drive the decision. The directive on paper was a compressed version of those values. Asking the family to tell you who the person was is often how you reach the living version of the directive.

19.6 Another Real Example

Meet Elena. She was a palliative care nurse at a memory care unit. Her patient was Mrs. Ofori, an 88 year old woman with end stage dementia. Mrs. Ofori had a directive from 2010 stating no feeding by artificial means if she became unable to feed herself.

Mrs. Ofori had stopped being able to feed herself two years ago. Her family and the facility had continued hand feeding her small amounts. She seemed to enjoy it. Now she was developing recurrent aspiration. The facility medical director wanted the family to consider stopping hand feeding. The daughter, Aisha, was distraught.

Elena met with Aisha. She did not start with the directive. She said, "Tell me what your mother is like now. When you visit, what do you notice?"

Aisha said, "She smiles when I come in. She closes her eyes when the music plays. She eats the applesauce but coughs on the water. She opens her mouth when the aide comes with the spoon. She doesn't know I'm her daughter, but she knows I am someone she likes."

Elena said, "So you are with someone who is present, in some way, and who is still responsive."

Aisha said, "Yes. But the doctor says she might aspirate."

Elena said, "That is a real risk. What do you think your mother would say about that risk, if she could say anything?"

Aisha thought for a long time. She said, "I think she would say, 'If eating is one of the last things that brings me pleasure, I want to keep eating, even if there is risk.'"

Elena said, "That fits what you have told me about her. She loved food. She loved being at the table with family."

Aisha nodded.

Elena said, "The directive she wrote was about not wanting tubes. What you are describing is not tubes. It is comfort feeding. It comes with some risk. The directive doesn't really speak to this specific question. You and I have to think about what she would say about this specific situation."

Aisha said, "I think she would choose the eating."

Elena said, "I think I agree with you. Let's do a plan that keeps the comfort feeding going, with some precautions to reduce aspiration, and accept the risk as part of what brings her pleasure."

They did. Mrs. Ofori died six weeks later. She had eaten with pleasure until the last week. Aisha was at peace with the decision.

What this means for you: Directives usually speak to broad categories (tubes, hospital, CPR), not to the specific questions that come up in real care. When the directive does not quite fit, the move is to translate the directive back to its underlying values and then apply those values to the current situation. Aisha's mother was not asking about hand feeding in 2010. The clinician's job is to figure out what she would have said about hand feeding now, based on who she was.

19.7 FAST And The Hospice Conversation

The FAST scale, developed by Reisberg in the 1980s, is used to stage Alzheimer's disease progression (Reisberg, 1988). It consists of seven stages, with stage 6 and stage 7 broken into sub stages. Stage 7a indicates severe dementia, with the patient having very limited speech (approximately six or fewer intelligible words per day). For hospice eligibility under the Medicare benefit, patients typically need to reach FAST stage 7a or higher, plus have associated complications like aspiration, pressure sores, or significant weight loss.

The FAST is specifically validated for Alzheimer's disease. For other dementias (Lewy body, vascular, frontotemporal), clinicians use FAST as a rough guide supplemented by clinical judgment about disease trajectory and complications.

The FAST is clinically useful. It is also a conversation tool. When a family is trying to understand where their loved one is, the FAST stages give them a map. Instead of saying "your mother is in advanced dementia," you can say, "based on what I am seeing, your mother is at FAST stage 7b. She can no longer speak in full sentences, she needs help with all activities of daily living, and she is having difficulty with swallowing. This is a stage where hospice becomes appropriate."

The map orients the family. It tells them where they are. It also tells them what is likely ahead, though not on any specific timeline. Families who have seen the FAST often say later that the map was the single most useful thing they received, because it converted a vague sense that their mother was "getting worse" into a clear understanding of where she was and what was coming.

One caveat. The FAST was not designed to be a predictor of time to death. Many patients at FAST 7a or higher live for months or even years, particularly if they do not develop complications. Using the FAST to say "she has six months" is a misuse of the tool. Using it to say "she is at a stage where hospice care would be appropriate to support her quality of life" is accurate.

In MI terms, introducing the FAST works through elicit-provide-elicit. You ask the family what they understand. You share the FAST information briefly, with permission. You ask what they make of it. Families often have insights about their loved one's stage that even the clinical assessment missed. "I noticed she stopped using my name about six months ago" is a clinical observation. "She started being unable to feed herself last year" is another. The family's knowledge and the FAST framework together usually produce a shared understanding.

19.8 When It Does Not Work

The most common failure in dementia care conversations is applying the directive mechanically. The clinician reads the paper, draws the conclusion, and delivers it to the family. The family feels bulldozed. They resist not because the conclusion is wrong but because the process was not collaborative. Decisions that should have been easy become fights.

Three things to try:

1. Never open a decision conversation with the directive. Open with the patient. Ask the family to tell you who she was. Build the picture. When you eventually bring in the directive, bring it in as one piece of information, not as the verdict. 2. When the directive and the current situation diverge, say so out loud. "This document was written in 2012. It was not written about this specific situation. I want us to think together about what your mother would say about this specific thing." The acknowledgment of the gap makes space for real thinking. 3. When the family is stuck, ask them to tell you what their loved one would say. This is different from asking what they think should happen. It is asking them to channel the patient. Most families can do this, especially after you have helped them tell stories about who the patient was. Their channeling is often more reliable than their personal preference, because it carries the weight of decades of knowing the person.

A second failure is underestimating the patient's present responses. Some clinicians, trained to see advanced dementia patients as "not really there," miss the cues that they are. The patient who opens her eyes when a grandchild enters the room is telling you something. The patient who grimaces when moved is telling you something. Ignoring these cues produces decisions that might look logical on paper but that miss what the patient is actually experiencing.

19.9 The Quick Version

Dementia care at the end of life requires holding two standards at once: substituted judgment (what would the person have wanted) and best interest (what is most likely to promote wellbeing now). Both matter. When they match, decisions are clearer. When they differ, the family and the clinical team do the hard work of weighing.

The family's memory is often the richest source of the patient's voice. Elicit stories about who the person was. Listen for the orienting patterns. Let the directive be one piece of evidence, not the verdict.

Non verbal cues from the patient are real communication. Facial expression, response to music and familiar voices, feeding behavior, vocalization, body positioning. These cues are admissible in the clinical conversation. Formal tools like the PAINAD scale can discipline observation.

When past and present disagree, resist the urge for an easy answer. Look for the stronger, more stable signal. Bring the family in to help weigh. Honest acknowledgment of the gap often produces better decisions than mechanical application of either standard.

The FAST scale gives families a map. Introduce it through elicit-provide-elicit. Use it to orient rather than to predict. Hospice conversations are easier when the family has a shared picture of where their loved one is in the disease course.

The next chapter moves to the other end of the age spectrum. Pediatric palliative care has specific demands, and the MI skills you have built need to be adapted for children who are dying, for their parents, and for their siblings.

Chapter 20: Children Facing The Unthinkable

Amara had been a pediatric palliative care nurse for eleven years. She had been in the room for hundreds of conversations that nobody should ever have to have. On a Thursday afternoon in October, she walked into a room on the pediatric oncology floor to meet a 10 year old boy named Diego. Diego had relapsed neuroblastoma. The most recent trial had not worked. His oncologist had told his parents the previous day that there were no more curative options.

The parents had asked Amara to help them figure out how to tell Diego.

Amara sat down next to Diego's bed. Diego was playing a game on a tablet. His parents sat in the corner, their hands tightly clasped.

Amara said, "Diego, I am Amara. I am a nurse who helps kids who are really sick. Your mom and dad wanted me to meet you. Can we talk for a little bit?"

Diego paused his game. He said, "Are you here because I'm not going to get better?"

The room stopped. Amara did not lie. She also did not rush. She said, "That is a very important question. Tell me what you already know."

Diego said, "I know the medicine didn't work. I heard Dad crying in the hall last night. He doesn't usually cry. I think that means it's bad."

His mother started crying silently in the corner. His father put his arm around her.

Amara said, "You are right that the medicine didn't work. What do you want to know?"

Diego said, "Am I going to die?"

Amara said, "I think you probably are, yes. The doctors do not have any more medicine that will make the cancer go away."

Diego nodded slowly. He looked at his parents. He said, "Mom, don't cry. I knew already."

Then he looked back at Amara and said, "When?"

Amara said, "The doctors are not exactly sure. They think probably weeks to a few months. Some kids surprise everybody. We don't know for sure."

Diego said, "Okay." He was quiet for a moment. Then he said, "Will it hurt?"

Amara said, "We will work very hard to make sure it doesn't. We have good medicine for pain. Nobody wants you to hurt."

Diego said, "Where will I be?"

Amara said, "Where do you want to be?"

Diego said, "Home. With my dog."

Amara said, "Then that is where we are going to work to have you be."

The whole conversation took twelve minutes. Diego went back to his game afterward. He died at home seven weeks later, in his own bedroom, with his dog, Cheeto, curled at his feet and his parents on either side of him.

This chapter is about the work of pediatric palliative care. You will meet developmental considerations in eliciting children's values, learn to navigate parents as both gatekeepers and grievers, think about when and how to include siblings, understand the language children use for death and dying, and face the hardest question: what to do when a child's wish contradicts a parent's plan.

20.1 Developmental Considerations

Children are not small adults. Their understanding of death, their capacity to express preferences, and their emotional processing all depend on where they are developmentally. Elicit values work in children requires adapting the MI skills you already have to developmental stages.

Very young children (under 3) do not have a conceptual understanding of death as permanent. They do, however, have a clear sense of if they feel safe, if a caregiver is present, and if something hurts. Their values communication is largely non verbal. A skilled pediatric clinician watches what the child reaches for, what they turn away from, and who they calm down around.

Preschool children (3 to 6) often understand death as temporary or reversible. They may ask questions like "when will I come back" or "will I still get Christmas presents." Their emotional states are vivid and often short. They can tell you what they want to do today. Asking about weeks or months in the future is usually not useful at this age. The values that matter are immediate: being with mom, having their favorite toy, not being in pain right now.

School age children (7 to 12) often have a more developed concept of death. They understand permanence, though they may still have magical thinking ("if I am very good, maybe I will get better"). They can reflect on their own experience, can express preferences about the present and near future, and can often tell you what matters to them. Diego, at 10, was in this range. He could hold the conversation. He could ask questions. He could express his wishes clearly.

Adolescents (13 and up) often have a fully adult understanding of death. Their developmental tasks, though, complicate the picture. Adolescents are working on identity, autonomy, and peer belonging. A teenager facing death often has specific concerns that younger children do not: fairness, meaning, legacy, unfinished romantic relationships, friends who are going on to lives the teenager will not have. Their values elicitation often needs to include these concerns, which adults sometimes miss.

The clinical implication is that the questions you ask must match the child's developmental stage. To a preschooler, you might ask, "What makes today a good day? What makes it a bad day?" To a school age child, you can ask more future oriented questions, as Amara did with Diego. To a teenager, you often need to ask about meaning, peer relationships, and what they want to leave behind.

One constant across ages: children are often more willing to talk about their own dying than adults expect. Research on pediatric palliative care suggests that children who are able to ask direct questions about their illness and have them answered honestly report less anxiety and less distress than children whose parents and clinicians avoided the topic (Kreicbergs et al., 2004). The protection adults try to provide by not discussing death often produces more distress, not less.

20.2 Parents As Gatekeepers And Grievers

In pediatric palliative care, the parents are always in the room, literally and figuratively. They are the legal decision makers. They are also the people losing their child. They are simultaneously the gatekeepers of information to their child and the grievers of the future that is being taken from them.

This dual role creates specific challenges. Parents often want to protect their child from hard information. They think their child is "not ready" to know. They want to hold onto hope in front of their child, even when the hope is gone. Some parents instruct the team not to tell the child the diagnosis. Some parents want conversations to happen, but only on their terms.

The work with parents requires holding both dimensions.

For the gatekeeper dimension: parents do have legitimate authority about what and how their child is told. Their wishes carry weight. At the same time, research and clinical experience both support the child's right to information they are asking for. When a child asks a direct question, answering honestly is usually better than deflecting. The parent's protective instinct is real, but it often does not serve the child.

The move with parents is not to override their authority. It is to help them see that their child is already picking up on more than they think. Most children facing serious illness know something is wrong well before they are told. They hear the crying in the hall. They notice the silence when they walk into rooms. They feel the weight in their parents' hands. Keeping them uninformed often means keeping them alone with their unnamed fears rather than genuinely protecting them.

A useful conversation with parents:

"I want to talk with you about what Diego already knows, and what he might be wondering. My experience is that kids pick up on a lot more than we think. What have you noticed him saying or asking?"

"Would you be open to letting him guide what we talk about? If he asks, I will tell him honestly. If he doesn't ask, I won't bring it up. Is that something you could live with?"

"I know this is the last thing you want to talk to him about. You have been protecting him since the day he was born. Letting him have this conversation is also a form of protection. Different kind. But it is protection."

These conversations are hard. They often involve tears. They are worth doing, because they usually produce an agreement that lets the child have the conversation they need without violating the parents' authority.

For the griever dimension: the parents are also drowning. The anticipatory grief of losing a child is one of the most profound human experiences. They need support. They need to be seen. They need someone to acknowledge that what they are facing is unbearable. If the clinical team only engages with them as decision makers, and not as grieving humans, the decisions they make will be compromised.

A move that helps: set up some time with parents that is not about decisions. Just about them. "How are you holding up, right now, in this?" Invite them to say what they are carrying. Reflect. Do not try to fix. The conversation is not about producing a plan. It is about acknowledging that they are a person, not a decision making entity.

20.3 Sibling Inclusion

The siblings of a dying child are often the most neglected members of the family. The sick child gets the team's attention. The parents get some support. The siblings are often at school, or at a relative's house, or trying to stay out of the way.

Their experience is specific. They are losing their brother or sister. They are also watching their parents transform in ways that are unfamiliar and frightening. They are trying to navigate school and peers while carrying something that nobody at school understands. They often feel they have become invisible.

The research on sibling outcomes after the death of a child is sobering. Siblings of children who died of cancer report higher rates of anxiety, depression, and post traumatic stress than peers for years afterward (Sveen et al., 2018). Factors that are protective include being included in conversations about the illness, being given accurate information, and feeling that their own experience was acknowledged by the adults around them.

Concrete ways to include siblings:

Ask the parents if the siblings have been involved in conversations. If not, offer to meet with them.

Meet with siblings at their developmental level. A 7 year old does not get the same conversation as a 15 year old.

Ask siblings what they already know and what they are worrying about. The worries they have are often not what the adults assume.

Give siblings a role, if they want one. Sitting with the sick sibling. Reading to them. Playing quiet music. Bringing a favorite toy. Roles combat the feeling of being useless.

Acknowledge their grief directly. "Your sister is very sick. That is hard. You are allowed to feel everything you are feeling. You are allowed to still want to go to soccer practice. You are allowed to be angry at her for being sick. All of it is okay."

Help the parents see the siblings. Parents in the grip of their sick child's illness sometimes lose track of the healthy ones. A team member who asks, "how are [sibling names] doing with this?" can remind the parents that there are other children who also need them.

After the death, the siblings need continued attention. Bereavement support should include them, not just the parents.

20.4 The Language Children Use

Children talk about death in their own ways. Clinicians who work with children learn to listen for the specific vocabulary, metaphors, and indirect approaches that children use.

Young children often use concrete images. "When I die, will there be bugs?" "Is it going to be cold?" "Do dead people sleep?" These questions sound strange to adults. They are the child's way of working out a concept they do not yet have words for. The response is to answer honestly and concretely. "When people die, their bodies stop working. They do not feel cold because they cannot feel anything. Some people believe that a part of you continues somewhere else. I don't know what happens for sure, but I know the people who love you will always love you."

Older children and adolescents often approach death through fiction or reference. They may bring up a movie, a video game, a book character who died. This is often a way of talking about their own death at a safer distance. Taking the reference seriously, and then gently connecting it to their own situation if they want, can open the conversation.

Some children talk about their death in the third person or in hypotheticals. "What if a kid my age died. What would happen?" This is not avoidance. It is the child giving themselves a way to explore the topic without committing to it. Following their lead, staying in their frame, often produces more useful conversation than insisting on directness.

Some children will refuse to talk about death at all. That is also data. The refusal is sometimes developmental, sometimes about protecting the parents, sometimes about not being ready. Respect it. "You do not have to talk about it if you do not want to. When you do want to, I am here."

One specific move. Ask children about their dreams. Many children with serious illness have vivid dreams that surface what they are processing. "Have you had any weird dreams lately? What have they been like?" The answers are often rich, and they give the clinician access to the child's inner life without requiring the child to do abstract emotional work.

20.5 A Real Example

Meet Omar. He was a pediatric social worker at a children's hospital. His patient was a 14 year old girl named Layla with advanced osteosarcoma. The disease had spread to her lungs. Her prognosis was weeks to months.

Layla's parents had been in the hospital with her for three weeks. They had not told her the prognosis. Her mother, in particular, was insistent that Layla "not be told." Her father was quieter, but deferred to her mother.

Omar met with the parents first. He said, "Tell me about Layla. What is she like."

The parents talked for twenty minutes. About how she loved art. About how she was sarcastic. About how she was close to her younger brother Raj. About how she had been writing a novel for the last year.

Omar said, "She sounds like someone who is very aware and who pays attention."

Her mother said, "She is."

Omar said, "What is she asking you right now about what is happening?"

Her mother said, "She keeps asking if the new treatment is working. We keep telling her we will know soon."

Omar said, "You are telling her what feels safest for you to tell her."

Her mother cried.

Omar said, "What do you think she would want to know, if she could choose?"

Her mother was silent. She said, "I think she would want to know. She has always wanted to know."

Omar said, "I agree. And I think the longer she does not know, the more alone she is going to feel."

Her mother said, "I can't tell her."

Omar said, "I can be with you while you tell her. I can help. But I think this is a conversation that needs to happen, and I think it is better coming from you than from anyone else."

The next day, the parents told Layla. Omar was in the room. Layla cried. She said she had known. She said she had been waiting for someone to say it. She asked her parents to stop pretending. She said she wanted to finish her novel and read it to her brother. She had six weeks left. She finished the novel. She read it to Raj the week before she died.

What this means for you: Parents who want to withhold information from a dying child are almost always acting out of love. They are also, almost always, leaving the child alone with what the child already knows. Helping the parents see this, with compassion, is often the move that lets the real conversation happen. The parents do not need to be overridden. They need to be supported in doing the hard thing they know they need to do.

20.6 Another Real Example

Meet Fatima. She was a pediatric palliative care physician in her ninth year. Her patient was a 12 year old boy named Marcus with end stage cystic fibrosis. Marcus was in the hospital. His lungs were failing. His mother wanted him on a ventilator. Marcus did not.

Marcus had told the respiratory therapist, in a quiet moment, that he did not want to be intubated. He said he had seen what it looked like from his time in the CF community. He said he was tired. He said he wanted to go home.

His mother did not believe this was really his wish. She thought the RT had misheard, or that Marcus was saying what he thought the RT wanted to hear. She demanded that the ventilator be ready.

Fatima convened a meeting with Marcus, his mother, and his father. She asked Marcus if he would be willing to tell his parents, directly, what he wanted. He said yes.

She prepared him. "What do you want to say to them?"

Marcus said, "That I don't want the ventilator. That I know what it means. That I want to go home."

In the meeting, Fatima supported Marcus while he spoke. His mother wept. She said, "You do not understand what you are saying. You are a child."

Marcus said, "Mom, I have been sick my whole life. I know what I am saying. I am tired."

Fatima said to the mother, "You are hearing your son, who has been sick his whole life, tell you what he wants. His voice in this is real. He is at the stage developmentally where he can hold this. He has been in the CF community his whole life. He has seen it. He knows."

The father said to the mother, "Let him have this."

The mother collapsed into her husband. She said, through tears, "I can't lose him."

Fatima said, "You are losing him. The question is how he gets to say goodbye."

They brought Marcus home. He died there four days later, without being intubated, on his own terms, with his mother holding him.

What this means for you: The child's wish, when it contradicts the parents', is not automatically overridden. A 12 year old with chronic illness has often thought about their own dying in ways most adults have not. Their expressed preferences, when they are clear and stable, deserve weight. The clinician's job is not to decide for the parents or for the child. It is to make sure the child's voice is heard, that the parents understand what they are hearing, and that the decision that is made is one the child can live with, even if only for a few more days.

20.7 When A Child Contradicts A Parent

The hardest pediatric palliative cases are when a child's expressed wishes contradict the parents' plans. These cases are rare but real. Most often they involve adolescents who have clear capacity to express preferences about their own care.

Legally, parents retain decision making authority for minors in most jurisdictions. But "retain authority" is not the same as "unilaterally override." Courts, ethics committees, and clinical teams have long recognized that adolescents' expressed preferences carry weight, especially in end of life decisions (Committee on Bioethics, 2016).

The move when a child and parent disagree is not to choose sides. It is to ensure the child's voice is heard clearly, that the parents understand what they are hearing, and that everyone involved is making decisions with full information.

Specific steps:

Assess the child's capacity. Does this child understand what is being decided, the likely consequences, and the alternatives? Adolescents over 12 often do. Younger children sometimes do, for decisions that are developmentally accessible.

Separate the child's voice from the parents' interpretation. Sometimes parents, especially under distress, hear what they fear rather than what the child said. Meeting with the child alone can surface the child's actual views.

Help the parents hear the child. Not "your child is right and you are wrong." Something like: "I want to make sure you hear what he is saying, because he is saying it clearly, and I think you might be filtering it through your own fear."

If the disagreement persists, involve ethics consultation. Ethics committees are there for exactly this kind of situation. They are not there to override the family. They are there to help the family, the clinical team, and the child's voice all be heard.

Be honest about what the law allows. In some cases, parents' authority will prevail even when the child disagrees. In those cases, the clinical team should still ensure the child's voice is documented and considered, even if the final decision goes against the child's expressed wish.

Above all, do not let the disagreement become about winning. The goal is not to prove someone right. The goal is care that serves the child, respects the family, and allows everyone to have as good a death or as good a final period as possible.

20.8 When It Does Not Work

The most common failure in pediatric palliative care is adult centered communication. The team talks with the parents. The parents talk with each other. The child is off to the side, on a tablet, or sleeping, or staring at the ceiling. The child is often the most aware person in the room. The child is rarely included.

Three things to try:

1. Involve the child. Every visit, ask the child something directly. Not just about their symptoms. About their day, their favorite thing, their worries, their wishes. The child learns that they are a participant, not an object of discussion. 2. Respect the child's cues. If the child does not want to talk today, honor that. If they want to play a game while you talk with the parents, let them. Their presence is what matters. Full engagement is not required every time. 3. Bring other team members with specific skills. Child life

specialists, pediatric chaplains, and art or music therapists can often reach children in ways that medical staff cannot. These professionals are not adjuncts. They are central.

A second failure is underestimating what children know. A 6 year old who has been in the hospital for months knows much more about their illness than adults assume. Asking them what they think is happening is often revealing. Telling them what is happening, rather than asking, often produces worse conversation than asking first.

20.9 What To Take Away

Pediatric palliative care requires adapting the MI skills you have to the developmental stage of the child. Very young children communicate values non verbally. Preschoolers focus on the immediate. School age children can hold future oriented conversations. Adolescents have adult level understanding complicated by adolescent developmental tasks.

Parents are both gatekeepers and grievers. They have legitimate authority. They also often underestimate what their child already knows. The work with parents is to hold both roles: honor their authority, acknowledge their grief, and help them see that their child is usually more aware than they think.

Siblings are often neglected. They need to be seen, included in conversations, given roles if they want them, and supported through bereavement. Their outcomes depend on being treated as central, not peripheral.

Children talk about death in their own ways. Through concrete images, through fictional reference, through third person hypotheticals, through refusing to talk at all. Following their lead, rather than insisting on directness, usually produces better conversation.

When a child's wish contradicts a parent's plan, the move is not to choose sides. It is to ensure the child's voice is heard, that the parents understand what they are hearing, and that the decision is made with full information. Adolescents' expressed preferences carry weight, especially in end of life decisions, even when parents retain legal authority.

The next chapter moves to a different dimension of context. Cultural considerations shape every conversation in palliative care. Chapter 21.0 is about holding cultural humility as a default posture, asking about disclosure preferences early, treating collective decision making as legitimate, working effectively with interpreters, and recognizing spiritual care as part of clinical care.

Chapter 21: Culture Shapes Every Conversation

Mrs. Wei was 71 years old and had been a restaurant owner in a Chinese American community in San Francisco for thirty one years. She had been diagnosed with pancreatic cancer. Her oncologist, Dr. Kim, had just received the staging results. The cancer was locally advanced and metastatic. The prognosis was approximately six months.

Dr. Kim had planned to meet with Mrs. Wei and her family to share the results. Before the meeting, her oldest son Ming asked to speak with Dr. Kim privately.

Ming said, "Doctor, I want to ask you something. In our culture, we do not tell the patient the diagnosis if it is fatal. My mother will give up if she knows. We would like you to speak with the family, and then we will decide what to tell her. Can you respect that?"

Dr. Kim was Korean American. She had seen versions of this request before. She also felt the tension in it. Her medical training emphasized patient autonomy. American bioethics had been built on the principle that the patient has the right to know their diagnosis. Withholding information from the patient, on its face, violated that principle.

She also knew that her training had been shaped by a specific cultural context (Euro American, individualistic) that was not universal. Many cultures treat medical decision making as a family matter rather than an individual one. Many cultures view direct disclosure of terminal diagnoses as harmful to the patient. What looked like paternalism through one lens was protection through another.

Dr. Kim said, "Ming, thank you for telling me that. I want to understand what you are asking for. Can you tell me more about how this usually works in your family?"

Ming explained. The family would receive the information. They would gather with elders and decide what to tell Mrs. Wei, how to tell her, when, and how much. They would protect her from anything that would cause her despair. They would make decisions about treatment together. Her role, in their understanding, was to be cared for, not to be burdened with the full weight of the diagnosis.

Dr. Kim said, "I hear you. I want to do this in a way that honors your family's wishes and also respects your mother. Can I ask something? What if I spoke with your mother first, just for a few minutes, and asked her what she wants to know? She might tell me directly that she wants her family to know and not her. That is something she is allowed to do. Or she might tell me she wants to know. Either way, it would be her own wish. Would that work?"

Ming was quiet. He said, "I think that would be acceptable. If she tells you to give the information to us, you will do that?"

Dr. Kim said, "Yes."

Dr. Kim met with Mrs. Wei briefly. She said, through an interpreter, "Mrs. Wei, we have results from your tests. Before I share them, I want to ask you something. Some people want to know everything about their health. Some people prefer that their doctor share information with their family, who will decide what to tell them. What works for you?"

Mrs. Wei smiled gently. She said, in English, "My son will tell me what I need to know."

Dr. Kim said, "That is what you want?"

Mrs. Wei said, "Yes. My son is a good son. He knows me."

Dr. Kim spoke with the family. The family, with Ming taking the lead, decided to tell Mrs. Wei that her illness was serious but not to use the word "terminal." They made treatment decisions collectively. Mrs. Wei died four months later, at home, surrounded by her family, having participated in the aspects of her care that she wanted to and having been protected from the aspects she did not want.

Dr. Kim later said, "I learned that respecting autonomy does not always mean direct disclosure to the patient. Sometimes autonomy is exercised by delegating. What mattered was that Mrs. Wei herself told me what she wanted."

This chapter is about that work. You will meet cultural humility as a default posture, learn to ask about disclosure preferences early rather than assuming, understand collective decision making as a legitimate form of autonomy rather than an obstacle, learn to work effectively with interpreters, and recognize spiritual care as clinical care.

21.1 Cultural Humility

Cultural competence has long been taught as a framework in healthcare. The idea was that clinicians could learn the preferences, beliefs, and practices of different cultural groups and apply that knowledge in care. The framework has real uses. It also has real limits.

The limits are that culture is not a checklist. A Chinese American family may or may not follow traditional Chinese disclosure practices. A Latino family may or may not hold collective decision making as central. An Orthodox Jewish family may or may not be strict about withdrawal of treatment. Assuming you know what someone wants because of their background is a different kind of stereotyping, even when dressed up as competence.

Cultural humility is a different orientation (Tervalon and Murray Garcia, 1998). It is the posture that you do not know, that you need to ask, that each patient and family is an individual within whatever cultural frame they bring. It is the recognition that your own cultural frame is not universal, and that what looks like deviation from the norm is often just deviation from your norm.

In practice, cultural humility looks like asking questions you might otherwise assume answers to.

"Tell me about your family. Who are the people who make decisions with you about your health?"

"Are there things that matter to you about how medical information gets shared?"

"Are there religious or spiritual practices that are important in how you want to be cared for?"

"Are there things I should know about your family's traditions around illness and dying?"

These questions do not require you to be an expert on any particular culture. They require you to approach the patient and family as the experts on their own culture, and to adapt accordingly.

One important note. Cultural humility does not mean accepting every request as equivalent. A family practice that endangers the patient, or that violates the patient's own expressed wishes, may need to be declined. But most of what cultural humility uncovers is not conflict with clinical ethics. It is difference in expectation that can be accommodated once it is understood.

21.2 Asking About Disclosure Early

One of the highest leverage moves in culturally humble palliative care is asking about disclosure preferences at the beginning, before any bad news has to be delivered.

"Before we get to the results of your tests, I want to ask you something. Some people want me to share everything directly with them. Some people prefer that I share information with their family, and their family decides what to tell them. What works for you?"

"We have not yet gotten to the point where we are sharing difficult information. I want to make sure I understand your preferences now, so I get it right when the time comes. Are there things I should know about how you want to receive medical information?"

"As things evolve, I may have information that is hard to hear. Different families handle that differently. Can you tell me what would be most helpful for your family?"

Asking this early accomplishes several things. It signals that you are not assuming a default. It gives the patient the opportunity to express autonomy by either requesting direct disclosure or delegating it. It prevents the awkward scenario of discovering disclosure preferences only after you have already said something the family wishes you had not.

The research on disclosure preferences across cultures shows substantial variation (Goldberg, 1984; Rosenberg et al., 2017). Many patients from traditions that emphasize collective decision making prefer that family members be informed first. Other patients from the same traditions prefer direct disclosure. The only way to know is to ask.

A related move. When a family requests that information be withheld from the patient, do not automatically agree or automatically decline. Explore what the request is really asking for, as Dr. Kim did with Ming. Often the request can be accommodated in a way that also respects the patient's own autonomy, by offering the patient the choice of who receives information.

One caution. If the patient has expressed preferences for direct disclosure and the family is requesting that you withhold, the patient's preferences prevail. The patient's autonomy includes the right to delegate to the family. It does not extend to the family's right to override the patient's own expressed wishes. Navigating this requires tact. You honor the patient's preference while acknowledging the family's concern, often through separate conversations where the family's grief and worry can be addressed without shifting the decision.

21.3 Collective Decision Making

Much of bioethics training treats individual autonomy as the default, with collective decision making framed as a departure from the default. This framing is not culturally neutral. In many cultures, collective decision making is the default, with individual decision making seen as strange, isolated, or even disrespectful to family.

A Latino family that meets to decide together. A Chinese family where the oldest son leads. A South Asian family where elders are consulted. An African American family where the church community participates. An Orthodox Jewish family where the rabbi is involved. None of these is an obstacle to autonomous decision making. They are different forms of autonomous decision making, in which the patient's autonomy is exercised within and through a collective rather than in isolation from it.

Treating collective decision making as legitimate, rather than as an obstacle, changes the way you run conversations.

You ask who should be in the room, rather than assuming the patient alone.

You plan for decisions to take time, because the collective process is slower than individual decision making.

You provide information that can be shared within the collective, rather than insisting on one patient centered conversation.

You respect the role of specific family members (oldest son, eldest daughter, designated elder) who carry authority within the system.

You accept that the patient may genuinely want the family to decide, rather than interpreting this as deference or passivity.

One useful reframe for clinicians who have been trained individualistically: the patient who says "whatever my family decides" is not necessarily being passive. They may be exercising a cultural form of autonomy in which their preference is precisely that the family be involved. Honoring that preference is honoring their autonomy, not overriding it.

The difficulty comes when the collective is not unified, when family members disagree, or when the patient's individual wishes seem to differ from the family's decision. In those cases, the work of Chapter 17.0 applies. You reflect each perspective. You find shared values. You locate the patient's own voice and help it be heard within the family process. The framework is the same as for any family conflict, with the added recognition that the family process itself is legitimate, not something to be bypassed.

21.4 A Real Example

Meet Isabella. She was a hospice nurse in a community that served many Spanish speaking patients. Her patient was Mr. Diaz, a 78 year old man with end stage heart failure. His family was extensive: wife, six children, seventeen grandchildren, three siblings. His wife and oldest daughter were the primary caregivers.

Isabella, who was not Latina, asked in her first visit, "Mr. Diaz, who in your family makes decisions with you about your health?"

Mr. Diaz said, "My wife. And my oldest daughter. They talk together. Then they ask me. Then we decide."

Isabella said, "So all three of you together."

He said, "Yes."

Isabella made a practice of ensuring all three were present at every significant conversation. When she could not get all three, she would communicate with the ones present and ask them to share with the missing one before any decision was made. This took longer than individual decision making. The family appreciated it.

When Mr. Diaz developed a pneumonia and the question of hospitalization came up, Isabella did not ask Mr. Diaz alone. She said, "I want to talk with you, your wife, and your daughter together. Can we set up a time?"

They met. Mr. Diaz said, "I don't want to go to the hospital."

His wife said, "He does not want to go."

His daughter said, "Papa, are you sure?"

He said, "Yes, mija. I am sure."

His daughter said, "Okay."

The decision was made through the family, with Mr. Diaz at the center. Isabella supported the process. Mr. Diaz died two weeks later, at home, with his wife, his six children, and most of the grandchildren present. His wife told Isabella later, "You understood us. Some of the other nurses wanted to talk to him alone, like he was a lone man. He was never alone. That was what he loved about his life."

What this means for you: Collective decision making is not something to work around. It is something to work with. Patients whose families are central to their identity experience family inclusion in decisions as a respect for who they are. Bypassing the family, even in the name of patient autonomy, can feel to the patient like being separated from the people who matter most.

21.5 Working With Interpreters

Many end of life conversations happen across languages. The quality of the conversation depends heavily on the quality of the interpretation. This is a clinical skill that is often underdeveloped.

The first rule: use a professional medical interpreter whenever possible. Not a family member. Family members interpreting for their own loved ones carry the weight of the diagnosis as they translate. They also often soften or edit, either to protect the patient or to protect themselves. Professional interpreters are trained to interpret accurately, to stay in their role, and to maintain a position of neutrality that family members cannot.

The second rule: address the patient directly, not the interpreter. Even though the words come out in a different language, you are talking to the patient. Look at them. Pause after each thought to let the interpreter interpret. Wait for the response. Do not say, "Tell her that I said..." Say, "Mrs. Gomez, I want to share some results with you."

The third rule: pace yourself. Speak in short, clear units. After each unit, stop and let the interpreter work. Resist the temptation to deliver long paragraphs that then have to be remembered and translated. Short units are easier to translate accurately and easier for the patient to absorb.

The fourth rule: allow time. Conversations through an interpreter take longer. Double the time you would budget for a conversation in a shared language. If you feel rushed, either reschedule or accept that the conversation will not finish in one session.

The fifth rule: check for understanding. After a key piece of information is interpreted, ask the patient to tell you in their own words what they heard. "Mrs. Gomez, I want to make sure I communicated this clearly. Can you tell me, in your own words, what you heard?" The interpreter will interpret her response. This gives you a check on how the message landed.

Some specific challenges are worth naming.

Some languages do not have direct equivalents for certain medical or emotional terms. The word for "hospice" does not exist in every language. The word for "prognosis" may not map cleanly. Work with the interpreter before the meeting, if possible, to understand how terms will be translated.

Some cultures consider direct discussion of death taboo. The language used matters. Rather than "your mother is dying," some families respond better to "she is very sick" or "she may not recover." The interpreter can often advise on this.

Some patients may switch between languages. A bilingual patient may prefer to speak in one language about some topics and another about others. Follow their lead. Do not assume that because they speak English fluently, they want the hard conversation in English.

One last note. Family members sometimes insist on interpreting. "My mother trusts me. She won't talk to a stranger." Acknowledge this, and then offer a compromise. "I understand. Let's have the professional interpreter here as well, just so the medical parts are accurate. You can be in the room. You can talk to your mother yourself. The interpreter is there for precision, not to replace you." Most families accept this when it is explained kindly.

21.6 Another Real Example

Meet Hassan. He was a palliative medicine physician at a large urban medical center. His patient was Mrs. Abdullah, a 72 year old Somali woman with metastatic breast cancer. She did not speak English. Her family spoke both Somali and English. The hospital had Somali medical interpreters on staff.

The first meeting was with the family only. Her oldest son, Omar, asked if the team could interpret through him rather than using the professional interpreter. Hassan said, "I want to honor your request. I also want to tell you something. When we use a professional interpreter for medical conversations, it lets you be in a different role. You can be her son, listening with her, grieving with her. You do not have to carry the weight of delivering the words yourself. Would you be willing to try it with the interpreter, and you can be her son in the room?"

Omar agreed reluctantly.

The interpreter, a woman named Zara, met with Hassan before the family conversation. They talked about how to translate specific medical terms. Zara told Hassan that in Somali culture, death was typically discussed in indirect terms, and that she would soften some of the medical language while staying accurate. Hassan agreed.

In the conversation with Mrs. Abdullah, Hassan spoke in short units. He paused after each. Zara interpreted. Mrs. Abdullah asked questions through Zara. Hassan could tell from her face that she was tracking the conversation, not just the words.

At one point, Mrs. Abdullah said something in Somali. Zara interpreted: "She says, 'I know. Allah has written it. I am ready.'"

Hassan paused. He said, "Tell her I hear her. Tell her that what we will focus on now is making sure she is comfortable, that she is at home with her family, and that her last weeks honor who she has been."

Mrs. Abdullah smiled through tears. She reached for Omar's hand. The conversation shifted to practical planning.

Afterward, Omar said to Hassan, "Thank you for using Zara. My mother said things to her she would not have said to me. It was better this way."

What this means for you: The professional interpreter is not a workaround. They are an enabling presence. They let the family member be present as a family member, rather than being the conduit for hard information. They also bring cultural competence that a physician from a different background cannot bring. When you use an interpreter well, the conversation is better, not just possible.

21.7 Spiritual Care As Clinical Care

In many cultures and traditions, the spiritual dimension of dying is not separate from the medical dimension. A Muslim family who wants to orient the patient's bed toward Mecca in the final hours is not doing something "extra" to the medical care. They are doing something that is as important to them as the medical care. A Catholic patient who wants last rites is not asking for something outside of clinical purview. The last rites are part of what a good death looks like to them.

Treating spiritual care as clinical care means integrating it into the plan, not relegating it to an afterthought.

Specific moves:

Ask about spiritual preferences at admission. Not just the formal question ("what is your religion"), but the functional question ("are there spiritual or religious practices that are important to how you want to be cared for, especially near the end?").

Involve chaplains early. Hospice chaplains are trained in both clinical pastoral care and in working across religious traditions.

They can be with patients whose traditions are different from their own.

Respect specific practices. Dietary restrictions, timing of prayer, preferences about who can be present at the death, specific rites that must be performed. Build these into the care plan.

Do not assume that a patient's religious tradition is the same as their actual practice. A Catholic patient may be devout or non practicing. A Muslim family may be strict or liberal. Ask what the specific patient and family want, not what you expect based on their stated tradition.

Recognize that spiritual care also applies to patients who are not religious. "What gives your life meaning? What would make these last weeks feel right to you?" are spiritual questions. They can be answered in religious or non religious frameworks.

The research on spiritual care in end of life is strong. Patients who report that their spiritual needs are supported by the medical team have better quality of life scores and better bereavement outcomes for their families (Balboni et al., 2010; Phelps et al., 2009). This is not an add on. It is part of effective palliative care.

One note about clinician comfort. Some clinicians feel awkward engaging in spiritual conversations. They do not share the patient's tradition. They do not feel qualified. That is a reasonable concern, and it is why chaplains are on the team. But the basic move (asking what matters, listening, reflecting) does not require you to share the patient's tradition. It requires you to be present with them in whatever tradition or non tradition shapes their dying.

21.8 When It Does Not Work

The most common failure in culturally responsive palliative care is assuming rather than asking. The clinician, with good intentions, applies what they think they know about a particular culture and gets it wrong, because this patient is not the generic patient of that culture. Or the clinician, with the best intentions, avoids asking because they fear offending, and then misses what the patient actually wants.

Three things to try:

1. Ask, do not assume. The question "tell me what is important to your family in how we do this" is almost always welcomed. It signals respect. It gives the patient and family the chance to share what you need to know. 2. If you make a cultural mistake, acknowledge it. "I realize I did not ask about your family's traditions around this before I said what I said. I am sorry. Can you tell me more about what would be helpful for us to do?" Acknowledging the mistake usually repairs the relationship better than pretending you did not make one. 3. Work with interpreters and chaplains as partners, not as support staff. They bring expertise that you do not have. Consulting them before and during conversations produces better care. Failing to involve them often produces care that is technically adequate but culturally off.

A second failure is treating cultural difference as an obstacle to "real" bioethics. Some clinicians, faced with a family that wants to withhold information from a patient, experience this as a conflict with autonomy rather than as an expression of a different understanding of autonomy. Working through this requires humility about what autonomy means, and willingness to find accommodations that honor both principles rather than insisting on one.

21.9 Where You Are Now

Cultural humility is different from cultural competence. It is the posture of not knowing, of asking, of treating the patient and family as experts on their own context. It prevents the stereotyping that can come from assuming you know what a cultural background means for a specific patient.

Asking about disclosure preferences early gives the patient the chance to express autonomy through choice rather than through forced disclosure. Some patients want to know everything. Some want family to be informed and to decide what reaches them. Both are legitimate exercises of autonomy when the patient has made the choice themselves.

Collective decision making is not an obstacle to autonomous decision making. It is a different form of it, in which the patient's preferences are exercised within and through a family or community rather than in isolation. Respecting the collective process means slowing down, ensuring the right people are in the room, and honoring the roles that different family members carry.

Working with interpreters is a clinical skill. Use professionals. Address the patient directly. Pace yourself in short units. Double the time. Check for understanding. Work with the interpreter before the meeting when possible. Let family members be present as family rather than as conduits.

Spiritual care is clinical care. Ask about practices. Involve chaplains early. Respect specific rites and dietary requirements. Do not assume a patient's tradition based on stated affiliation. Engage the spiritual dimension even for patients who are not religious, through questions of meaning and value.

With Part V complete, the book turns to the sustainability of the clinician who does this work. Part VI begins with a chapter about your own grief, which is as real as the grief of the families you work with, and which has been accumulating for as long as you have been doing this.

PART VI: SUSTAINING YOUR PRACTICE

Chapter 22: Your Own Grief Matters Too

Gemma had been a hospice nurse for twelve years. She was good at her job. She was known on her team as someone who stayed calm in the hardest situations, who could guide families through the worst hours, who always had the right reflection at the right moment. She had been asked, three times, to give talks at regional conferences about her work.

On a Tuesday evening in March, Gemma came home from work, set down her bag, took a glass of water to the kitchen table, and sat down. Her husband asked how her day had been. She said, "Fine." She drank her water. She looked at the kitchen wall.

Then she said, aloud, to no one in particular, "I think that was the eight hundred and forty seventh."

Her husband said, "The eight hundred and forty seventh what."

Gemma said, "Patient I have seen die."

She sat with the number for a while. Then she said something that surprised her. "I don't think I have grieved any of them."

She cried for the first time in years. Not performatively. Not the quiet professional tears she sometimes allowed herself with families. A real, bent over at the table, heaving kind of cry.

This chapter is about the grief that Gemma was finally touching. You will learn about **secondary loss** and **cumulative grief**, the practices of **reflective practice** that prevent the accumulation Gemma was carrying, how to do **peer supervision** in a way that actually helps, how to think about **boundaries** in home based hospice work, and the question of when to step back from this work and how to do that well.

22.1 Secondary Loss And Cumulative Grief

Clinicians who work in end of life care experience a specific kind of grief that has several names in the literature: secondary loss, professional grief, compassion fatigue, cumulative grief. The phenomenon is real, understudied, and often ignored in training.

Secondary loss refers to the grief that accumulates when you lose patients and families you have grown close to, even though your relationship with them was professional rather than personal. You did not have the deep history that a spouse has with a dying person, but you had weeks or months of real relationship. The loss is smaller than family loss, and it is not zero. Over time, small losses accumulate into something substantial.

Cumulative grief refers to the weight of multiple losses carried together. A clinician who loses one patient can grieve that patient. A clinician who loses fifty patients over a year does not get to grieve each of them. Most of the deaths become part of a blur. The cumulative effect is different from the sum of individual griefs. It produces numbness, dissociation, a sense of going through the motions, and, eventually, physical and emotional symptoms.

Compassion fatigue and **burnout** are related but distinct. Burnout is exhaustion from workload and systemic failure. Compassion fatigue is specifically the depletion of the emotional resource that lets you care for other people's pain. Cumulative grief often contributes to both.

The research is clear. Hospice and palliative care workers report high rates of compassion fatigue, burnout, and elevated rates of depression and anxiety compared to general healthcare workers (Pereira et al., 2011; Whitebird et al., 2013). The contributing factors are not just the volume of deaths. They are the quality of attention the work requires. Hospice work is emotionally saturated. Showing up for families in their worst hours, over and over, takes a toll that is different from clinical work that is mostly technical.

Naming what is happening is the first step in working with it. Gemma's recognition at the kitchen table was not a breakdown. It was a breakthrough. The grief had been there for twelve years. It had been waiting for her to make space for it.

22.2 Reflective Practice

The clinical response to cumulative grief is reflective practice. This is a term that has been so overused in healthcare that it has become background noise. Let me be specific about what it means and how it works.

Reflective practice is the regular, deliberate process of stopping to think about the work you are doing. Not thinking about how well you did it. Thinking about what is in you after doing it.

It has a few forms.

Journaling. Writing down what happened in a visit or with a patient. Not charting. Journaling. The chart captures the clinical facts. The journal captures what you carried out of the room. A five minute entry at the end of a day can keep grief from accumulating unprocessed.

Debriefing. Talking with a colleague after a hard case. Not formally. Not in rounds. Just "that was a lot, I need to say some things about it out loud." Having someone who will listen without needing to fix it is precious. Being that person for someone else is part of the work.

Ritual. Some clinicians develop small rituals after a patient's death. A moment of silence. Writing the patient's name. Lighting a candle at home. Sending a note to the family. These rituals mark what happened rather than letting it slide past.

Supervision. More formal than debriefing. Regular time with a supervisor or peer supervisor where you bring difficult cases and work through what they brought up in you. Supervision is essential in mental health training. It is essential in hospice work too, though it is rarely provided.

The common feature of all these forms is that they create time and space for the work to settle rather than accumulate. The losses still happen. They just do not get stored in a place where they compound.

One specific practice. Some hospice teams hold periodic memorial meetings where they name the patients who have died in the last period and say something brief about each one. Not clinical. Personal. "Mrs. Kowalski loved the same song as my grandmother." "Mr. Afolabi told me a joke I still remember." These meetings do not take long. They do what needs doing: they acknowledge that these were people, not just cases, and that the clinicians carry something after each one.

22.3 Peer Supervision That Works

Much of what passes for peer supervision in hospice settings is actually case review. The team gets together, discusses a clinical case, decides what to do next. That is useful for care planning. It is not supervision.

Real peer supervision is different. It is time set aside, with one or more trusted colleagues, specifically to work on what the work is doing to you. The focus is not on the patient. It is on the clinician.

The structure that often works:

A small group (three to five people), meeting regularly (every two weeks to every month).

A time boundary (60 to 90 minutes).

A ground rule of confidentiality.

A focus on reflection, not problem solving.

Rotating attention, so each session is focused on one person's experience.

A facilitator who is trained in this kind of work, or a group that has built the skills over time.

The content is different from case review. "I want to talk about a visit I had on Tuesday. The patient was actively dying and the family was fighting in the kitchen. I went home and could not sleep. I want to work out why." That is supervision. Not because the question has a clinical answer, but because naming the why is what lets the clinician move through it.

Groups that work together over time develop a kind of trust that lets them go deeper than surface talk. A clinician who has been in a peer supervision group for two years will share things they would not share anywhere else. They will cry. They will name things they are ashamed of. They will receive compassion and challenge from people who have earned the right to offer both.

Without this kind of support, many clinicians develop coping patterns that protect them short term and damage them long term. Emotional numbing. Workaholism. Distancing from their own families. Substance use. Cynicism. These patterns are not signs of personal weakness. They are predictable responses to cumulative loss without adequate processing. Prevention is supervision.

If your team does not have a peer supervision structure, consider starting one. If formal supervision is not possible, pair up with one colleague and commit to regular phone or in person check ins. The structure matters less than the consistency. What sustains clinicians over time is having places where they can be seen in the cost of the work, not just in the competence of it.

22.4 Boundaries In Home Based Hospice

Home based hospice has a specific challenge that inpatient work does not. The clinician is in the patient's home, in their intimate space, sometimes for months. Relationships become more personal than they typically do in hospital or clinic settings. The boundaries that are easy to maintain in a clinical office blur in a kitchen.

Some of the blurring is good. A nurse who becomes a trusted presence in a family's home during the hardest time of their lives is doing work that is inseparable from the relational texture of home based care. The personal quality of the relationship is part of what helps.

Some of the blurring is not good. Clinicians who become emotionally enmeshed with patients and families can lose the capacity to act clinically. They can find themselves working off the clock, taking on responsibilities that are not theirs, carrying emotional burdens that belong to the family rather than to them. The costs compound.

Practical boundaries for home based hospice work:

Time boundaries. Be clear about when you are working and when you are not. Most hospice agencies have on call structures for a reason. Use them. Do not give patients your personal cell phone number. Do not respond to calls from families during your off hours unless it is a true emergency within your scope.

Role boundaries. You are the nurse, the social worker, the chaplain, the aide. You are not the friend, the family member, the unpaid caregiver. Families sometimes try to pull you into roles that are not yours. Gentle redirection is part of the work. "I care deeply about your mother. My role is to be her nurse, not her friend. The friend role needs to come from the people in her life. I can help connect her to those people."

Emotional boundaries. You can be moved by a patient's situation. You cannot carry their grief as if it were your own. The distinction is sometimes subtle. Supervision helps you stay on the useful side of it.

Physical boundaries. Home visits have a time window. Beyond that window, you leave. Families sometimes want you to stay longer. "I wish I could stay. I have to get to my next visit. I will be back on Thursday." Saying this without apology is a skill. Families often understand it better than clinicians expect.

Gift boundaries. Many families offer gifts of appreciation. Food, small items, cash. Agencies typically have policies. Know them. Hold them kindly. "I cannot accept cash gifts. The cookies, thank you." Accepting small food gifts is usually fine. Accepting larger gifts can cross into dual relationships that compromise care.

Post death boundaries. After a patient dies, the relationship with the family changes. You may or may not continue contact. Most hospice agencies have formal bereavement programs. Use them. Personal ongoing relationships with bereaved families are usually not recommended, because they blur the professional role and may not serve either the family or the clinician well.

These boundaries are not rigid walls. They are the structure that allows the relational work to be done sustainably. Clinicians who have no boundaries burn out within a few years. Clinicians who have too many boundaries become distant and less effective. The craft is in the middle.

22.5 A Real Example

Meet Amara. She was a hospice chaplain in her fifteenth year of work. She had been carrying a sense for about eighteen months that something was wrong. She was not sleeping well. She was more irritable at home. She had stopped calling friends. She was eating in ways she had never eaten before.

She spoke with a colleague who was a mental health professional. The colleague asked her what was happening at work. Amara talked for an hour. About patients. About families. About what she had seen.

Her colleague said, "When was the last time you grieved a patient's death, on purpose?"

Amara said, "I don't think I have, honestly. Not since the early days."

Her colleague said, "I think that is what is happening."

Amara started journaling. She wrote about each death, at the end of the week. She also joined a peer supervision group that met monthly. She began a personal practice of lighting a candle at home after each death.

Within three months, her sleep improved. Within six months, she felt more present at home. The irritability eased. The eating settled into a better pattern. She was still doing the same work. She was just letting the work settle rather than accumulate.

A year later, she said to her colleague, "I had been numb for years without knowing it. The journal and the group gave me back to myself. I am a better chaplain now because I am allowed to be present with my own grief rather than only with other people's."

What this means for you: The accumulation happens gradually. The recovery also happens gradually. Structures that let you process as you go (journaling, peer supervision, small rituals) are what prevent the situation from getting to where Gemma's was at the kitchen table. If you are already there, the work is still possible. It just takes more deliberate attention.

22.6 Another Real Example

Meet Marcus. He was a palliative medicine physician in his eleventh year. He had built a program from nothing. He was respected. He was also, by his own later admission, on the edge of leaving medicine entirely.

Marcus had three small children. His wife, a teacher, had been telling him for a year that he was not present when he was at home. He had been dismissing her concerns as her not understanding the demands of the work. When she finally said, "You are here but you are not here, and I don't know how much longer I can do this alone," he heard her.

He called a colleague and asked if they could talk. The colleague, a geriatrician in her twentieth year, listened. She said, "Marcus, when did you last take more than three consecutive days off work."

Marcus could not remember.

She said, "I did the same thing for the first eight years. I almost lost my marriage. I stopped because I realized I was not going to be able to do this work for another thirty years at that pace."

They talked about what she had changed. She had taken on a supervisor who checked on her regularly. She had protected her weekends. She had stopped accepting every referral. She had started a daily meditation practice. She had made peace, slowly, with the fact that good enough was the goal, not perfect.

Marcus took her advice. He cut his hours. He hired an additional physician for the team. He started going to his kids' games. He took a real vacation for the first time in years.

Two years later, he was still in the work. His wife was no longer contemplating separation. His kids noticed he was more present. The program continued to do well, maybe better, because Marcus was more sustainable in it.

What this means for you: Some of the grief we carry as clinicians is about the life we are not living with our own families and friends while we are serving other families in their dying. This is not only about processing individual patient losses. It is about protecting the life that is ours. Sustainability in this work depends on having a life outside of it that is full enough to hold you.

22.7 When To Step Back

Sometimes the work becomes unsustainable. The signs are specific.

Physical symptoms that do not resolve. Persistent sleep problems, persistent gastrointestinal issues, persistent headaches, weight changes, chronic exhaustion.

Emotional symptoms. Irritability that is disproportionate. Numbness. Dissociation. Difficulty feeling anything.

Behavioral signs. Substance use that is increasing. Withdrawal from relationships. Avoidance of work tasks that used to be manageable.

Cognitive signs. Intrusive thoughts about patients outside of work hours. Difficulty concentrating. Clinical judgment that feels off.

Any of these on its own is a yellow flag. Several together is a red flag. Red flags mean you need help. Help can be therapy, supervision, time off, or a change in the scope or intensity of your work.

Stepping back is not failure. It is stewardship. A clinician who takes three months off and returns is more valuable than a clinician who works through until they have to leave the field entirely. Many of us have been trained in cultures that treat endurance as the highest virtue. In this work, endurance without care is often the path to losing yourself.

If you step back, step back with structure. Take real time off. Not "catching up on admin" time. Real off. Tell your team what you are doing. Accept help. Consider therapy if you have not. When you return, return slowly. Set new boundaries. Do not fall back into the old pattern.

Some people leave the work permanently, and that is also not failure. Some of us are called to this work for a season. Others are called to it for a career. Either is honorable. Forcing yourself to stay past your season produces a clinician who is present in body but gone in spirit, and that is not a gift to the patients.

22.8 When It Does Not Work

The most common failure in self care for hospice clinicians is treating it as a checklist. Yoga on Sunday. Journaling twice a week. Peer supervision monthly. The checklist can feel like another performance of adequacy, another thing to do perfectly, another way of measuring yourself.

Three things to try:

1. Start with one thing. Not a plan. One thing. Five minutes of journaling before bed. One phone call with a colleague after a hard case. One scheduled boundary around weekends. Build from there. Most sustainability practices that last start small. 2. Attend to the body. Cumulative grief lives in the body. Sleep, movement, nourishment, and connection with people who love you are the foundation. No psychological practice works if these are neglected. 3. Find one person who will tell you the truth. A friend, a colleague, a therapist, a supervisor. Someone who will say, "You sound like you are not doing well" when you are not doing well, even when you are telling everyone else that you are fine. The honest mirror is one of the most protective things you can have.

A second failure is isolation. Clinicians in this work sometimes feel that their experience is unshareable, that their friends who are in other fields will not understand. Some will not. Some will, more than you think. And other hospice and palliative care clinicians definitely will. Do not be alone with what you are carrying.

22.9 Where You Are Now

This work accumulates. Secondary loss and cumulative grief are real phenomena that produce real symptoms over time. Naming them is the first step in working with them. Ignoring them produces the Gemma at the kitchen table moment, which comes for most clinicians eventually if the work goes unprocessed.

Reflective practice is what prevents accumulation. Journaling, debriefing, ritual, and formal supervision all play a role. The specific form matters less than the consistency. Clinicians who process as they go do not carry what clinicians who do not process as they go carry.

Peer supervision is different from case review. It focuses on the clinician, not the case. It requires trust, confidentiality, and regular time. Where formal supervision is not available, paired check ins with a trusted colleague are a reasonable substitute.

Boundaries in home based hospice are not walls. They are the structure that makes relational work sustainable. Time, role, emotional, physical, gift, and post death boundaries all matter. Clinicians who have none burn out. Clinicians who have too many become distant. The craft is in the middle.

Stepping back is stewardship, not failure. Signs to watch for include persistent physical symptoms, emotional numbness or dissociation, behavioral changes, and cognitive difficulties. When these appear, help is needed. Time off, therapy, supervision, or a change in scope can all be part of the response.

The final chapter of Part VI is about taking what you have learned and building it into the team you work with. Good individual practice in MI and palliative communication is only part of the picture. A team culture that supports and reinforces these practices is what allows them to scale beyond what any individual clinician can do alone.

Chapter 23: Building An MI Team Culture

Dr. Yuki Tanaka had been the medical director of a midsize hospice program for six years. In that time, she had run three communication training initiatives. The first was a one day workshop in 2021 with an outside consultant. The team enjoyed the workshop. Nothing changed in practice afterward. The second was a series of monthly lunch and learns in 2022. Attendance dropped off after the third session. The third was a mandatory online module in 2023 that everyone completed and nobody remembered a week later.

In early 2024, Yuki sat down with her clinical educator, a nurse named Fatima, and said, "I keep trying to improve how our team communicates. Nothing sticks. What am I missing."

Fatima said, "Your trainings were good. You were treating it as a content problem. It is a culture problem. The skills need somewhere to land. We have been sending people to workshops and then returning them to a culture that does not practice what they learned."

They spent three hours mapping what a different approach might look like. They started a fourth initiative in 2024. It stuck.

The fourth initiative was not a training series. It was a slow redesign of how the team worked. MI skills were embedded in interdisciplinary rounds. Audio recordings were used for feedback that was not punitive. Role plays became a regular part of team time. Yuki herself started modeling the skills in the meetings she ran. The organization began tracking a few simple metrics that mattered to the team.

Two years later, the team was practicing differently. Family satisfaction scores had improved. Clinician retention had improved. The culture had shifted. Yuki said at a regional palliative care meeting in 2026, "I spent three years trying to change people one training at a time. What worked was changing the structure they worked in."

This chapter is about that structural change. You will learn how to embed MI in interdisciplinary rounds, how to build coding and feedback systems that support rather than punish, how to run role plays the team actually wants to do, the role of leadership modeling, and how to measure what matters without creating a bureaucracy nobody can sustain.

23.1 Embedding MI In Rounds

Most hospice and palliative care teams have some version of interdisciplinary rounds. Cases are reviewed. Plans are updated. Problems are raised. Rounds are efficient when they are focused on clinical content. They are also a place where team culture is either reinforced or eroded.

Embedding MI in rounds means changing some of what happens in the meeting.

Ask values based questions about every patient, not just the hard ones. "What matters most to this patient right now?" as a routine question in case review turns MI from an intervention for difficult cases into a baseline practice.

Share examples of specific moves that worked. "In the meeting with the Johnson family on Tuesday, I tried the double sided reflection when they were arguing about the feeding. I want to tell you what happened." This makes talking about craft routine rather than framing it as only about outcomes.

Name challenges without judgment. "I had a hard time with the Ortega family last week. I could not find the shared value. Anyone have thoughts." Inviting help on craft problems is different from case consultation. It signals that the communication work is work, that everyone gets stuck, and that help is available.

Rotate who leads. If the same person always runs rounds, the rounds reflect their style. Rotating leadership, even briefly, exposes the team to different approaches and prevents the rounds from becoming a performance for one leader.

Make time for the human in the case. At the end of a case discussion, a question like "how is this case sitting with you?" invites the clinician to share what they are carrying. This is not therapy. It is a minute of attention. Done routinely, it does more for team sustainability than any formal intervention.

The research on interdisciplinary rounds in palliative care supports a broad version of this approach. Teams that use structured communication tools and that explicitly discuss values and goals in their rounds produce care that is better aligned with patient preferences and report higher team satisfaction (Sanders et al., 2018).

One warning. Do not turn rounds into a training opportunity. If every case becomes an occasion for the leader to teach, the team will disengage. The goal is to embed the practice in the rhythm of the work, not to make every meeting a lesson.

23.2 Coding And Feedback

One of the most effective ways to develop MI skill is through coding. A clinician records a conversation (with consent), codes it using a tool like MITI 4, and gets feedback on their behaviors. Reflections counted. Questions counted. Reflection to question ratio calculated. Percent complex reflections calculated. These numbers are not a grade. They are a mirror.

The problem with coding in team settings is that it is often experienced as punitive. If the numbers are bad and they are shared with supervisors, clinicians may resist recording. If recordings are used in performance reviews, the whole process becomes about avoiding blame rather than learning.

For coding to work culturally, it needs to be:

Voluntary, at least initially. Clinicians choose to record and submit conversations for coding. Mandatory coding produces anxiety that interferes with learning.

Confidential. The raw data goes only to the clinician and possibly to a trusted coach. It does not go into personnel files. It is not used in evaluations.

Formative, not summative. The purpose is learning. Low numbers trigger conversation and support, not consequences.

Supported by training. Clinicians who have never been coded need orientation. They need to understand what the numbers mean and what good looks like. Without this, coding feels arbitrary.

Connected to goals the clinician has chosen. "I want to work on my complex reflections this month" is a different stance than "my supervisor told me my complex reflections need to improve." The first is self directed. The second is evaluative.

Sustainable. Coding every visit is unsustainable. Coding one visit per month, discussed in supervision, is sustainable.

The MITI 4 benchmarks for proficiency are specific (Moyers et al., 2016). Reflection to question ratio of at least 1:1. At least 40 percent of reflections should be complex. MI adherent behaviors above 90 percent. These benchmarks give clinicians something concrete to aim at. When approached as personal goals rather than as external standards, they can be motivating rather than deflating.

Some teams do group coding sessions. A recording is anonymized and played for the team. The team discusses what they notice. The clinician who was recorded gets feedback from multiple perspectives. The team learns collectively. Done well, this is powerful. Done poorly, it is humiliating. The difference is the culture of the group and the skill of the facilitator.

23.3 Role Plays The Team Wants

Role plays are the core of MI training. They are also what most teams resist. The reasons are specific. Role plays feel artificial. They feel like performance. Clinicians feel judged by peers. They feel they are being put on the spot. Many adults have not role played since some bad experience in nursing school or medical school.

Making role plays work for a team requires attention to several things.

Start small. A two minute role play of one moment, not a fifteen minute full scenario. The small size reduces the performance anxiety and gives everyone something achievable.

Focus on one specific skill. "Today we are going to practice complex reflections. Every time the patient says something, the clinician responds with a complex reflection. That is the entire exercise." This narrow focus makes the role play about skill building rather than about whole case performance.

Accept failure openly. Everyone messes up the first few times. The facilitator should model this. "I just tried a complex reflection and it came out wrong. Here is what I was going for. Let me try again." When the leader fails publicly and corrects, the room relaxes.

Use real scenarios, slightly modified. Made up cases feel fake. Modified versions of cases the team has actually seen land. "Let's do a version of the meeting we had last week with the family you know who was arguing. I will play the daughter." Clinicians who know the case can engage more fully.

Let people watch before they do. Observing a few role plays before taking a turn gives people a sense of what is being asked. It also lets them study what others do.

Rotate roles. The clinician sometimes plays the patient or family member. This is often the most instructive part. Being on the receiving end of a bad reflection or a rushed advance to content is educational in a way that performing the skills is not.

Include debrief. After the role play, ask the clinician: what worked, what was hard, what would you do differently. Ask the person who played the patient: how did you experience that. Short. Two to three minutes. This is where the learning consolidates.

Keep it regular. Role plays that happen once a year are an event. Role plays that happen every two weeks become part of the work. Regularity matters more than intensity.

Some teams resist role plays no matter what. For those teams, start with something less intimidating. A one hour facilitated case discussion where people describe specific moves they tried. Or pairs practice where two clinicians take five minutes to try a specific skill on each other. These smaller interventions can build toward role plays over time.

23.4 Leadership Modeling

The biggest determinant of how strongly an MI culture takes hold is the leaders practicing it. A medical director who lectures about MI in meetings but does not use it in their own practice produces a team that sees MI as rhetoric rather than behavior.

Modeling means doing the thing visibly. Specifically:

When you run a case review, ask values questions. "What did she tell you mattered to her." "What did the family say they were worried about." Over time, the team asks these questions too.

When you give feedback to your team, use reflections. "What I hear you saying is that you are frustrated because the family is not engaging." The feedback lands differently when it is reflected back rather than diagnosed.

When you yourself make a communication mistake with a family, name it. "I rushed that conversation. I wish I had slowed down. I am going to try again Thursday." Leaders who name their own craft failures give the team permission to name theirs.

When a team member shares a success, affirm specifically. "What you did with the Johnson family was a clean complex reflection in a high pressure moment. That worked because you had the patience to wait for it." Specific affirmations model the kind of affirmation you want the team to offer patients.

When you sit in on a difficult conversation, be present without taking over. Many medical directors, in family meetings, take over the room. A leader who sits back and supports the team member who is running the meeting is modeling something important.

The research on leadership and organizational change in healthcare is consistent. Initiatives that succeed have leaders who model the practices they are asking others to adopt (Damschroder et al., 2009). Initiatives that fail often have leaders who issue directives without changing their own behavior. The team reads the signal. What leaders do matters more than what they say.

One practical note. Leaders often do not know when they are not modeling. The behaviors that do not fit the espoused values are often invisible to the person enacting them. A trusted deputy who will tell you, "When you did X in the meeting, that was not MI," is essential. Receive the feedback. Adjust. Over time, the modeling becomes more consistent.

23.5 A Real Example

Meet Omar. He was the clinical supervisor of a home hospice agency in Colorado. He had inherited a team where communication practices varied widely. Some clinicians were excellent. Some struggled. There was no shared language.

Omar started with a single change. Every clinical team meeting, he added five minutes at the end where one team member would share a "moment from the week": a specific interaction they had with a patient or family that they wanted to reflect on. Not a clinical case. A moment.

The first few weeks, team members offered surface level moments. "The Johnson family seemed happy." Omar would gently ask follow up questions. "What specifically did you do that they responded to." Over time, the moments got richer.

After three months, Omar added a second change. One clinician per meeting would present a recording (with patient consent) of a short piece of a conversation. The team would listen. They would discuss what they heard. Not to critique. To learn.

The first recording was Omar's own. He played five minutes of a family meeting he had run. He said, "I want you to tell me what I could have done better. I am going to listen."

The team was tentative at first. Then one nurse said, "I think you missed an affirmation in minute three. She told you she had been taking care of her mother alone for four months. You said 'that is a lot' and moved on. You could have named specifically what she had been doing."

Omar said, "You are right. I missed it."

That moment, Omar later said, changed the culture. The team saw that the leader was willing to be coached. After that, clinicians started bringing recordings of their own. Within a year, the team had a shared language. Clinicians were practicing MI consistently. Family satisfaction scores had improved.

What this means for you: Cultural change often starts with the leader modeling vulnerability, not with the leader teaching skills. Omar's willingness to have his own recording critiqued in front of the team gave the team permission to do the same. The rest followed from that opening.

23.6 Another Real Example

Meet Aisha. She was the director of a hospital palliative care consult service. Her team consisted of three physicians, two nurse practitioners, two social workers, and a chaplain. She had been trying to integrate MI into the team's practice for two years with mixed success.

She decided to try a structured approach. She paired clinicians with each other for peer coaching. Each pair would meet for thirty minutes twice a month. They would listen to a short segment of one clinician's recorded conversation, and the other would give feedback. Then they would switch.

She also established a monthly group session where one pair would present their work to the whole team. Not to be evaluated. To share what they had learned.

The pairs were assigned across disciplines. A physician paired with a social worker. A nurse practitioner paired with the chaplain. This was uncomfortable at first. The chaplain said to Aisha after the first month, "I feel like I am not qualified to give feedback to a physician on her communication."

Aisha said, "You are exactly qualified. You hear things the physician does not hear. That is the point."

By month four, the pairs had settled. By month eight, the team's language had shifted. Doctors were talking about complex reflections. Nurses were noticing when their affirmations were generic. The chaplain was giving specific feedback on MI skills that she herself had not been trained in, because she had learned by listening carefully.

A year in, the team's family satisfaction scores had improved modestly. More importantly, the team's own satisfaction had improved. The chaplain told Aisha, "I feel more like part of the clinical team now. The peer coaching made me feel I had something to contribute."

What this means for you: Structural interventions like cross disciplinary peer coaching can build MI culture faster than more traditional training. The intervention also tends to flatten hierarchies and improve interdisciplinary respect, which is often undervalued in team effectiveness.

23.7 Measuring What Matters

Teams often resist metrics because metrics feel bureaucratic. The resistance is reasonable. Bad metrics drive bad behavior. Teams in hospice do not need a dashboard with thirty seven indicators that take an hour a week to report.

They do need a few simple signals that tell them if they are doing good work. The signals should be connected to what the team cares about, not to what administrators want to count.

Some signals that are worth tracking:

Family satisfaction with communication. Simple survey, one to two questions, delivered after admission and after death. "Did you feel your concerns were heard?" "Did you feel informed about what was happening?"

Clinician retention. How long do people stay. When they leave, do they leave to another palliative care position, or do they leave the field entirely. The second is a red flag about organizational health.

Use of peer supervision. Number of clinicians participating. Number of sessions held. Not every clinician will participate. Most should.

Percentage of patients with a documented goals of care conversation within 48 hours of admission. This is a process measure, but it tells you if the values first work is actually happening.

Coded fidelity for a sample of clinicians who choose to be coded. Voluntary, confidential, used for development.

Notice what is not on this list. Length of stay. Hospice enrollment rates. Cost per patient day. These are important to administrators and payors. They are not signals of MI culture. A team can score well on all of them and still be practicing badly.

The key is to keep the measurement simple and to use it for learning rather than for punishment. When scores drop, the response is curiosity, not blame. "What is going on that our family satisfaction scores dipped this quarter? Let's look at what has changed." This approach produces more learning than investigating individual clinicians.

Finally, do not measure what you do not plan to act on. If no one will look at the data, do not collect it. The act of collecting data that is not used teaches the team that measurement is for show, and that erodes trust in any future measurement effort.

23.8 When It Does Not Work

The most common failure in team MI initiatives is trying to change everything at once. A new protocol, new training, new metrics, new leadership expectations, all introduced in the same month. The team is overwhelmed. They comply performatively. Nothing sticks.

Three things to try:

1. Pick one thing. Change that one thing. Let it settle for three to six months before adding the next. Cultural change is slow. Trying to move faster usually produces less actual movement. 2. Involve the team in choosing the one thing. "What is the part of our communication practice that we most need to improve" is a better starting question than "here is what we are going to do." Teams that help design the intervention sustain it. 3. Celebrate small wins. When the team catches something (a clinician tries a new reflection that works, a family meeting that produced a good plan), name it out loud. Culture shifts partly through accumulated small positive feedback.

A second failure is leadership change. A new director arrives. They have different priorities. The MI initiative loses its sponsor. It withers. Protecting the work against leadership change requires embedding it in structures (peer coaching pairs, regular meeting practices, documented routines) that survive individual leaders.

23.9 What To Take Away

Team culture, not individual training, is what lets MI become practice. Most training initiatives fail because they return trained clinicians to cultures that do not support what was trained. The fix is not more training. The fix is redesigning the culture.

Embedding MI in interdisciplinary rounds makes values based questions routine rather than occasional. Coding and feedback work when they are voluntary, confidential, formative, and connected to goals the clinician has chosen. Role plays that the team actually does are small, focused, use real scenarios, treat failure as expected, and happen regularly rather than as occasional events.

Leadership modeling matters more than leadership training. Leaders who practice what they preach produce teams that practice. Leaders who give directives without changing their own behavior produce teams that comply performatively and learn nothing.

Measurement should be simple, tied to what the team cares about, and used for learning rather than punishment. A few signals (family satisfaction, clinician retention, peer supervision participation, documented goals of care conversations) are enough.

The closing chapter of the book is not about skills. It is about what all the skills are for. When you have been doing this work long enough, the skills disappear into something that is harder to name but more important than any individual technique. The next pages are about that.

Closing Chapter: The Conversation That Is Not A Technique

It was 4:17 a.m. The hospice chaplain, a man named Javier, sat in a chair next to the bed. His patient, Mrs. Haddad, was 79 years old, in the last hours of her life from end stage liver disease. Her breathing was shallow and irregular. Her eyes were closed.

Her daughter had been at the bedside for six days. She had finally gone to the hospital cafeteria for food, at Javier's gentle insistence, about twenty minutes ago. Javier had agreed to stay. The daughter had needed rest. Mrs. Haddad, who had spoken some English earlier in the week, was unlikely to wake again.

Javier was not doing anything that could be written in a clinical note. He was not using a reflection. He was not asking an open question. He was not introducing hospice services. He was not assessing for pain. He was not reflecting on the family's grief.

He was sitting there. His hand was resting lightly on Mrs. Haddad's hand. He was breathing slowly. Every minute or two, he was noticing the rhythm of her breath and letting his breath fall into it. The room was quiet. The sound machine was playing something that might have been ocean waves. The lamp in the corner gave a soft yellow light.

Javier was 62 years old. He had been a hospice chaplain for twenty three years. He had been in this specific moment, or moments enough like it to count, several thousand times. He was not thinking about what to do next. He was not rehearsing what to say when Mrs. Haddad died. He was not worried about if the daughter would get back in time.

He was just there. With her. In the quiet. In the last hour.

At 4:43, Mrs. Haddad took a slightly deeper breath and then did not take another. Javier noticed. He did not move his hand. He kept sitting. The monitor beside the bed did not beep because there was no monitor. He counted silently to sixty. No breath.

He stood up, kissed Mrs. Haddad gently on the forehead, and walked quietly to the nurses' station to call the daughter.

When the daughter arrived fifteen minutes later, she asked, "Was she in pain?"

Javier said, "No. She was peaceful. I was with her."

The daughter cried. Javier stayed with her for another two hours. He did not say much. He did not have to.

This is the closing chapter. Three short sections on what the book has been building toward.

Closing.1 When The Skills Disappear

Javier had every skill in this book. He knew how to do a complex reflection. He knew how to run a family meeting. He knew how to introduce hospice, how to talk about prognosis, how to roll with resistance when a daughter was refusing morphine at midnight. He had used those skills tens of thousands of times.

At 4:17 a.m., in the quiet room, none of those skills were visible. He was not performing any of them. He was just present.

This is what skilled practice looks like, in the end. The skills do not go away. They are absorbed into something that is harder to name. They become a capacity to be present, to pay attention, to meet whatever is in the room with what is in you. The skills were the training. The presence is the work.

Clinicians sometimes worry, when they are learning MI or any structured communication approach, that the technique will interfere with genuine connection. That concern is real at the beginning. When you are consciously trying to produce a complex reflection, you are not fully with the patient. You are watching yourself. The watching creates distance.

Over time, if you practice, the watching fades. The skills stop being things you are doing. They become things you do. You do not have to think about the reflection any more than you have to think about how to walk. You are still reflecting. You are just no longer constructing it. You are present, and the reflection emerges.

This is what Miller and Rollnick call MI spirit, or what other traditions call presence, or what some chaplains call ministry of presence. It is the same thing. It is what is left when the techniques have been practiced long enough to disappear into the practitioner.

You cannot skip to this. You have to go through the techniques. The early awkwardness of learning reflections, the performance of asking open questions, the self consciousness of practicing summaries. All of that is necessary. It builds the muscle memory that eventually lets the skills drop away.

Javier's twenty three years of chaplaincy were not wasted when he sat silently at Mrs. Haddad's bedside. Those twenty three years were why he could sit silently. A chaplain in their first year might have felt they needed to say something, to do something, to provide comfort. Javier had long since learned that his presence was the comfort. He did not need to produce anything else.

This is not mystical. It is craft. Any craft that is practiced long enough becomes embodied. The painter who has painted for forty years no longer thinks about brush technique. The surgeon who has operated for thirty years no longer thinks about incision angle. The clinician who has sat with dying people for decades no longer thinks about reflections. The skill is there. It is just no longer visible as skill.

Closing.2 What You Take Into The Next Room

You finish this book. You go back to work. Tomorrow or next week or next month, you walk into a room with a patient or a family or both, and you do not have the book with you. What you have is what has stayed with you.

What stays is not the specific techniques, though those matter. What stays is more like a disposition. A way of walking into the room.

A disposition to ask rather than assume what matters to the person in front of you.

A disposition to listen longer than feels comfortable before responding.

A disposition to reflect what you hear rather than advancing to what you want to say.

A disposition to check for understanding rather than hoping you got it right.

A disposition to hold ambivalence without trying to resolve it.

A disposition to let the family find their own yes rather than producing it for them.

A disposition to notice when you are rushing, when you are avoiding, when you are imposing, and to slow down.

A disposition to trust that the person in front of you knows things about their own situation that you do not know.

A disposition to be present to your own grief as a legitimate part of the work, rather than something to manage around.

These dispositions are what the skills were always pointing toward. The skills were scaffolding. The dispositions are the building.

You will not carry all of this into every room every day. Some days you will forget. Some days you will be tired and you will default to advice giving. Some days a family will push you and you will push back. That is fine. The work is not to be perfect. The work is to keep returning to the dispositions, over years and decades, until they are more of your default than the defaults you are trying to move away from.

One thing in particular to take with you. Every patient, every family, gets one version of their dying. Most of the people you will work with will die once, and their families will live with the memory of how it went for the rest of their own lives. What you do in those rooms matters in a way that most work does not. Not because you are saving anyone, you are not, but because you are present in a moment that will be remembered. The reflection you offer to a grieving daughter at 3 a.m. will be something she tells her own children about in forty years. The open question you ask an 82 year old man who has never been asked about himself will be something he thinks about in the last weeks of his life.

You do not get to know how it ripples. You can trust that it does.

Closing.3 The Invitation

This book ends with an invitation, not a conclusion.

Keep practicing. Not just the techniques, though yes, those. Keep practicing the larger thing. The attention. The presence. The willingness to be in the room with what is hard.

Find a peer supervision group, or a trusted colleague, or a therapist. Do not do this work alone. It is too much to carry alone.

Journal if that works for you. Light a candle if that works. Walk if that works. Make some practice of your own for noticing what you are carrying out of rooms, so that what you carry does not become what you are.

Read more. This book is one conversation. Miller and Rollnick's Motivational Interviewing is another. Atul Gawande's Being Mortal is another. BJ Miller's A Beginner's Guide to the End is another. Each of these voices will give you something different. The more voices you learn from, the richer your own voice will become.

Talk with your colleagues. The people you work with have seen things you have not seen. Ask them. Tell them what you have seen. Build the kind of team where the craft is discussed, the grief is acknowledged, and the practice can develop.

Care for patients and families. Care for yourself with the same seriousness. Those are not competing directives. They are the same directive. A clinician who attends to their own wellbeing can do sustainable work with patients. A clinician who burns themselves out for patients cannot, long term, be present for anyone.

And when you sit, at 4:17 a.m., next to a dying person you barely knew eight weeks ago, in a room that is quiet, with a lamp in the corner and a hand on a hand and no technique visibly in play, trust that you have been prepared.

All the reflections, the questions, the summaries, the affirmations, the hard conversations about hospice and prognosis and morphine and ventilators, the family meetings, the disagreements, the late arrivers, the dementia cases, the pediatric cases, the cultural negotiations, the team meetings, the training workshops, the failures, the recoveries, the years.

They are all present in the quiet. They are what let you be present in the quiet.

That is the work. It is the only thing the book was ever about. Everything else is preparation.

Appendix A: OARS Pocket Card

This card is for printing on a single double sided page (or a folded 4x6 card) and keeping in the pocket of a scrub top, a lab coat, or a clipboard. Nothing on this card will be new to you. It is a memory aid for the moments when you walk into a room and your mind goes blank.

A.1 Open Questions

Use open questions at the start of every visit. They invite a broad answer and cannot be answered yes or no.

For any first visit:

"Tell me about yourself, not just as a patient."

"What have you been told about your illness?"

"Who in your life knows what is happening?"

For the start of a follow up visit:

"How has this week been for you?"

"What has been on your mind since I saw you last?"

"What would be most helpful for us to talk about today?"

For values:

"What is most important to you right now?"

"What would a good day look like?"

"If things do not go the way we hope, what matters most to you?"

For caregivers:

"How are you holding up, really?"

"What is the hardest part of caring for him right now?"

"What do you wish the team understood about your situation?"

A.2 Affirmations

Affirmations name specific, observable effort or strength. Avoid "you are doing a great job" as a default. Too generic.

Better patterns:

"You learned how to [specific skill] in [specific time]. That is not something most people figure out that fast."

"You have been [specific action] for [specific duration]. That is harder than it looks."

"You noticed [specific thing] before anyone else did. You are paying attention to things most people would miss."

"You have been running on [actual amount of sleep] for [duration] and you are still [specific competent action]. That is taking something out of you."

When affirming ambivalence:

"You are weighing two things that both matter to you. That is not you being confused, that is you being careful."

"You are considering [option] and you are not ready to sign anything today. That tells me you are taking this seriously."

A.3 Reflections

Reflections capture what the speaker said, or implied, offered back. Target at least one reflection for every question you ask. At least 40 percent should be complex rather than simple.

Simple reflection pattern (repeats meaning in different words):

Speaker: "I don't know what to do." Reflection: "You are stuck."

Complex reflection pattern (adds meaning not explicitly spoken):

Speaker: "Everyone keeps telling me what to do." Reflection: "You are tired of being told, and you want someone to ask."

Reflection of feeling (names emotion directly):

"You are terrified that this is really happening."

"You feel relieved, and you feel terrible for feeling relieved."

"This is the worst thing that has ever happened to you."

Double sided reflection (holds both sides of ambivalence):

"You want him to keep fighting, and you also do not want him to suffer anymore."

"You know the chemo is not working, and you are not ready to stop."

Drop "it sounds like." Just say the thing.

A.4 Summaries

Summaries pull together what has been said, organize it, and hand it back. End with an invitation, not a conclusion.

Linking summary (connects to prior visit):

"When I was here Tuesday, you told me [specific content]. You also said [specific content]. How has that been since I saw you?"

Transitional summary (compresses a stretch of conversation before moving forward):

"Let me take a moment. You have told me [X]. You have told me [Y]. You have told me [Z]. Given those things, it makes sense to ask [next question]. Is that the conversation you want to have next?"

Collecting summary (in a family meeting):

"Let me try to say back what I have been hearing. [Name], you are saying X because Y matters to you. [Name], you are saying A because B matters to you. What I am hearing both of you agree on is that you love him and you want what is best. You disagree about what that looks like. Did I get anyone wrong?"

Always end with an invitation:

"What do you want to do with all of that?"

"Where do you want to go from here?"

"Is there anything I am missing?"

A.5 Quick Guide To Timing

Before medical content: open questions, affirmations.

During medical content: reflections, especially of feeling.

After medical content: pauses of seven to fifteen seconds, then reflections.

Before decisions: transitional summary, values questions.

End of visit: collecting summary, invitation to ask what has not been asked, specific next contact time.

A.6 Three Things Not To Do

Do not rush the pause after bad news. It will feel too long. It is not.

Do not fill ambivalence with a decision. Reflect both sides. Let the patient choose.

Do not answer a prognostic question with a number when a range would be more honest. "Weeks to a few months" is better than "six weeks."

Appendix B: Ten Scripted Scenarios With Annotated Responses

Each scenario below presents a short patient or family statement. Two possible clinician responses follow. The first is MI inconsistent. The second is MI consistent. Brief annotations explain why each lands the way it does.

These are not meant to be memorized or performed. They are meant to sharpen your ear for the difference between the two kinds of response, so that your own language moves toward the MI consistent side over time.

B.1 Scenario One: The Refusal Of Hospice

Patient, 68, with metastatic lung cancer, after his oncologist mentions hospice.

Patient: "I am not ready for that. That is giving up."

MI inconsistent: "Hospice is not about giving up. It is about comfort focused care that can actually add quality to your life. Many patients benefit from it. Let me explain what is involved."

Why this fails: The clinician has corrected the patient's framing without first understanding what the patient meant. The patient now has to choose between accepting the correction or defending their original view. Either way, the conversation is about a debate, not about the patient.

MI consistent: "Tell me what 'giving up' means to you, when you think about hospice."

Why this works: The clinician has treated the patient's statement as information rather than as a position to correct. The follow up question invites the patient to explain what they mean, which usually reveals a specific fear or memory that can be worked with. The conversation stays in the patient's frame.

B.2 Scenario Two: The Daughter's Plea

Daughter of a 79 year old woman with end stage dementia, after the hospice nurse suggests stopping the hand feeding that is causing aspiration.

Daughter: "I cannot be the one who starves my mother."

MI inconsistent: "You would not be starving her. In advanced dementia, the body no longer needs food the way it did before. Stopping hand feeding is not the same as starvation. There is good evidence that continued feeding at this stage does not extend life and can cause harm."

Why this fails: The clinician has led with medical facts in response to a statement of feeling. The daughter's statement was not an argument about physiology. It was a declaration that this specific act feels, to her, like something she cannot do. Facts do not move feelings.

MI consistent: "You have been feeding your mother her whole life. Stopping feels like stopping being her daughter."

Why this works: The reflection names what the daughter is actually experiencing. Once the feeling is named, the daughter often feels less alone with it. The medical facts may still be relevant later in the conversation. They will land better after the emotional ground has been acknowledged.

B.3 Scenario Three: The Late Arriving Son

Son of a dying mother, arriving from out of state after not visiting in eight months, in a family meeting on his first evening home.

Son: "Why is she not in the ICU? She should be getting everything possible. I do not understand why you are not doing more."

MI inconsistent: "Your mother has been on hospice for six weeks. She and your sister made these decisions together based on what your mother told us she wanted. The plan is not going to change now."

Why this fails: The clinician has defended the existing plan. The son is likely to hear this as being told he is too late to matter. He will either escalate or retreat in resentment. Either way, the grief underneath his demand has not been addressed.

MI consistent: "You got here last night. You walked in and saw your mother in a way that was very hard. You are now in a meeting where other people have been making decisions for months without you. That is a lot. I want you to know I see that."

Why this works: The reflection addresses what the son is actually carrying. It does not agree with his demand, and it does not dismiss it. It names his experience. From here, the conversation can move to what his mother told him over the years, which usually reconnects him to the existing plan without requiring him to capitulate to it.

B.4 Scenario Four: The Ambivalent Patient

A 62 year old woman with metastatic breast cancer, in a goals of care conversation about stopping chemotherapy.

Patient: "I want to keep trying. But I also do not know if I can keep doing this."

MI inconsistent: "It sounds like you are leaning toward stopping. Would it help if we talked about what a transition to comfort care might look like?"

Why this fails: The clinician has picked a side of the ambivalence and pulled the patient toward it. If the patient is not ready to be pulled, they will push back. If they are ready but being pushed, they may end up deciding to stop before they have fully arrived at that decision, which often produces regret.

MI consistent: "You want to keep trying, and you are also exhausted in a way that makes you wonder how much longer you can. Both of those are real, at the same time."

Why this works: The double sided reflection holds both parts of the ambivalence without privileging one. It tells the patient that her mixed feelings are normal. Once she feels she does not have to pick a side to please the clinician, she can actually think about what she wants. Decisions made from this ground hold better than decisions made under pressure.

B.5 Scenario Five: The Morphine Refusal

Wife of an actively dying 81 year old man, at 2 a.m. over the phone.

Wife: "I cannot give him the morphine. It will kill him."

MI inconsistent: "The morphine will not kill him. At the doses we use, it is safe. Please give him the dose. He is suffering."

Why this fails: The clinician is correct about the pharmacology. Pharmacology is not what is stopping her. She is not going to give the morphine after being told she is wrong. She is going to feel judged and become more paralyzed.

MI consistent: "You are afraid that if you give it, you are the one who ends him."

Why this works: The reflection names the actual fear. After this reflection, the clinician can move to sharing the pharmacology briefly. The wife will be more able to hear it because her fear has been acknowledged. If she still cannot administer the dose, the clinician can ask if someone else in the house can, which often resolves the paralysis.

B.6 Scenario Six: The Proxy Under Pressure

Oldest daughter, the designated healthcare proxy, after her brother has been loudly disagreeing with her decision to transition their father to comfort care.

Daughter: "I am starting to think I am making the wrong call. Maybe my brother is right."

MI inconsistent: "You are making the right call. Your father told you many times what he wanted. You are honoring that. Do not let your brother change your mind."

Why this fails: The clinician is being supportive, but in a way that makes the daughter's doubt feel wrong. Doubt in these situations is normal. Shutting it down does not resolve it. It just sends it underground, where it becomes harder to work with.

MI consistent: "Your brother is pushing back hard, and you are wondering if you are missing something. That is a real question worth sitting with. Tell me what your father told you, when he could still tell you, about how he wanted his last weeks to go."

Why this works: The clinician does not try to eliminate the doubt. They invite the daughter to check her decision against the patient's own words. If the decision holds up when she does that, the doubt resolves on its own. If it does not hold up, the decision needs to be revisited, and the daughter is in a better position to do that than to override her own concerns because the clinician told her to.

B.7 Scenario Seven: The Fearful Prognosis Question

A 58 year old man with advanced pancreatic cancer.

Patient: "Just tell me how long I have."

MI inconsistent: "I do not want to put a number on it. Every patient is different. Some live longer than expected. Some live shorter. We will focus on quality of life and see what happens."

Why this fails: The clinician has dodged the question. The patient asked for honest information. The evasion communicates that the clinician does not trust the patient with a real answer, or is not willing to take the risk of offering one. The patient is left with no usable information.

MI consistent: "Before I answer, can I ask what you would do differently with the information? That will help me give you the most useful answer. Then I will tell you what I think."

Why this works: The clinician invites the patient to say what they are trying to plan. The answer often reveals that the patient needs a rough order of magnitude, not a specific number. After the clarifying question, the clinician can offer a calibrated range ("weeks to a few months" or "months to a year") with an acknowledgment of uncertainty. The answer is usable without pretending to be more precise than it is.

B.8 Scenario Eight: The Estranged Spouse's Guilt

Husband of a dying woman whose marriage had been strained for years, sitting in the hospital corridor.

Husband: "I should have been a better husband to her. I don't know if I even have the right to be here now."

MI inconsistent: "You are here. You are doing the right thing now. Your wife knows you love her."

Why this fails: The reassurance does not land. He is carrying something real. Telling him that he is doing the right thing now does not touch the regret he is carrying about the years that he is not doing over.

MI consistent: "You are holding a lot of regret right now. You wish things had been different, and you are afraid that being here now is not enough."

Why this works: The reflection names the actual experience. Once it is named, he has something to work with. He may cry. He may say more. He may sit with it. Whatever he does next is his work, and naming the experience has made the work possible.

B.9 Scenario Nine: The Pediatric Parent's Request For Secrecy

Mother of a 12 year old boy with relapsed leukemia.

Mother: "Please do not tell him he is going to die. He is a child. He cannot handle it."

MI inconsistent: "Children often have a right to information about their own care. Research shows that children who are told the truth have better outcomes. I think we should tell him."

Why this fails: The clinician has led with an argument for disclosure. The mother is in anticipatory grief and trying to protect her son. Being lectured about research will not reach her. She will feel judged, not heard.

MI consistent: "You have been protecting him since the day he was born. The idea of telling him feels like you are breaking something. I understand that. Can I tell you what I have noticed over the years with kids his age? And then we can decide together."

Why this works: The reflection names her protective instinct as love, not as obstruction. The follow up invites her into a conversation about what the clinician knows, without making it a lecture. After she has been met, she is more able to consider the possibility that her son may benefit from being included, which is usually what eventually happens.

B.10 Scenario Ten: The Patient Who Does Not Want To Know

A 74 year old Chinese American woman, at a meeting where her family has told the physician they do not want her told her prognosis.

Patient: "My son will tell me what I need to know."

MI inconsistent: "I really think you should hear this directly from me. You are the patient. It is your right to know. Your son cannot decide what to tell you."

Why this fails: The clinician is trying to protect the patient's autonomy by overriding her actual expressed preference. Autonomy includes the right to delegate. By pushing direct disclosure, the clinician has ignored what the patient just said.

MI consistent: "You want your son to be the one who receives information and decides what to share with you. That is a real choice you are allowed to make. I will honor that. If at any point you want me to tell you something directly, you can tell me. Otherwise I will share what I know with your son."

Why this works: The clinician has respected the patient's chosen mode of engagement. The door is left open for her to change her mind. The patient has been treated as the agent of her own care, which is what autonomy actually means. The cultural practice of family mediated disclosure is honored without being imposed as a default.

Appendix C: The Serious Illness Conversation Guide With MI Overlays

The Serious Illness Conversation Guide (SICG), developed by Ariadne Labs, is the most widely used structured tool for serious illness conversations. This appendix walks through the guide section by section, adds MI overlays for each question, and flags where common MI mistakes happen in the structure.

The guide is a tool, not a script. Used well, it creates structure for a real conversation. Used poorly, it becomes a checklist that produces a series of answers without any of the understanding that matters.

C.1 Set Up The Conversation

SICG sets up by asking permission and explaining the purpose. The script typically includes language like: "I would like to talk about what is ahead with your illness and do some thinking in advance about what is important to you so that we can make sure we provide you with the care you want. Is this okay?"

MI overlay: This is an open invitation with permission seeking. Take it slowly. Wait for a real yes. If the patient hedges ("I guess so"), pause and check: "You sound a little hesitant. What feels uncertain about this?" Do not proceed into a serious illness conversation if the patient has not actually agreed to have one.

Common mistake: Racing through the setup because the clinician is nervous about the conversation. The setup sets the tone. Rush it and the rest will feel rushed.

C.2 Assess Understanding And Information Preferences

SICG asks: "What is your understanding now of where you are with your illness?"

MI overlay: This is an open question, and the right answer is whatever the patient says. Reflect what you hear. Do not correct. Do not add medical content yet.

Follow up reflections:

Patient: "I know the cancer has spread." Clinician: "You know the cancer has spread. You are thinking about what that means."

Patient: "They said this new treatment might help." Clinician: "You are hearing that the new treatment might help. You are hoping it will."

SICG then asks: "How much information about what is likely to be ahead with your illness would you like from me?"

MI overlay: This is the permission gate for prognostic sharing. Respect the answer. Some patients will want everything. Some will want limited information. Some will want information shared with family, not with them. All of these are legitimate.

Common mistake: Treating the response to this question as pro forma and then delivering prognostic information anyway. If the patient says "not today," do not share prognostic information today.

C.3 Share Prognosis

SICG offers language like: "I am worried that time may be as short as [weeks to months]."

MI overlay: Use calibrated ranges, not numbers. The "worried about" framing is useful because it acknowledges uncertainty while still being honest. Pause for seven to fifteen seconds after the prognostic statement. Do not fill the silence.

After the pause, reflect what you see: "That was a lot to hear." Or "You are somewhere else right now."

Common mistake: Following the prognostic statement with more content. Do not advance until the patient has had time to absorb what was said.

C.4 Explore Values And Goals

SICG asks a series of questions:

"If your health situation worsens, what are your most important goals?" "What are your biggest fears and worries about the future with your health?" "What gives you strength as you think about the future with your illness?" "What abilities are so critical to your life that you cannot imagine living without them?" "If you become sicker, how much are you willing to go through for the possibility of gaining more time?"

MI overlay: These are open questions that produce rich answers. The overlay is to resist moving to the next question when the current one has produced something substantial. Reflect. Ask follow up. Let the conversation expand.

Specifically:

When the patient names a goal, reflect it. "Being at your granddaughter's graduation in May matters more than anything else right now."

When the patient names a fear, reflect it. "You are afraid of dying in pain, like your father did."

When the patient names a source of strength, reflect it. "Your faith has carried you through before, and you are trusting it again now."

When the patient names an ability they cannot live without, check its stability. "Being mentally clear is so important to you that you would not want more time if it cost that. Is that right?"

Common mistake: Treating these as checklist questions and racing through them. The guide expects you to go deep on whichever question matters most to the specific patient. You are not obligated to ask all of them. You are obligated to reach what matters.

C.5 Close The Conversation

SICG suggests making a recommendation that is connected to the patient's stated values: "Given what is important to you, I recommend that..."

MI overlay: The recommendation works when it is genuinely grounded in what the patient has said, not when it is the clinician's preference dressed up in the patient's words. Before you make a recommendation, summarize what the patient said. "You have told me that being home matters most, that you do not want to suffer, and that you want to be clear headed for your grandchildren. Given those things, I would recommend [specific plan]."

End with permission to push back: "Does that feel right to you? What does not fit?"

Common mistake: Delivering the recommendation as a verdict. The recommendation should be a proposal that emerges from what the patient said, not a decision imposed from outside.

C.6 Document The Conversation

SICG provides a documentation template. Use the patient's own words where possible. A direct quote in the note is worth more than a paraphrase.

MI overlay: The documentation is part of the care. The note will be read by the clinicians who see the patient next. If the note is vague, the next clinician will have to reconstruct the patient's wishes from scratch. If the note has specific quotes and clear statements of priorities, the next clinician can honor what was established.

Template structure:

Illness understanding: [patient's words] Information preferences: [patient's stated preferences] Prognostic understanding shared: [what was said, and how the patient responded] Priorities: [specific, in order of importance] Fears: [specific] Sources of strength: [specific] Abilities the patient cannot imagine losing: [specific] Tradeoffs the patient is willing to make: [specific] Family knowledge: [who knows what, per the patient's report] Recommendation made: [what you recommended and why] Patient response: [how they responded: accepted, modified, or declined]

C.7 A Worked Example

Below is a condensed example of a conversation using the SICG with MI overlays, with the patient's words in quotes and the clinician's reflections and questions in plain text.

Setup.

Clinician: "I would like to talk with you about what is ahead with your illness and think together about what matters most to you, so we can make sure your care fits what you want. Is now an okay time?"

Patient: "Yes, I guess so."

Clinician: "I heard a little hesitation. What is coming up for you?"

Patient: "I am not sure I want to know what is ahead."

Clinician: "You are uncertain about how much you want to hear."

Patient: "Yes."

Clinician: "That is okay. We do not have to share everything I know. I can follow your lead on what would be helpful. Would it be okay to start by hearing what you are already understanding, and then you can tell me what you want to know and what you want to leave alone?"

Patient: "Okay."

Understanding.

Clinician: "What is your understanding now of where you are with your illness?"

Patient: "I know the cancer has spread to my liver. The last scan showed new spots in my lungs. My doctor said the chemo is not working as well as they hoped."

Clinician: "You know the cancer has spread. You know the chemo is not doing what you had hoped."

Patient: "Yes. I know I do not have a lot of time. I have not wanted to ask how much."

Information preferences.

Clinician: "Some people want to know about timeframes. Some people prefer not to. Where are you on that?"

Patient: "I think I would rather not know exactly. Just generally."

Clinician: "Okay. I can give you a general sense if it would help. We are not in a years time frame. We are somewhere in the months range. I could be wrong in either direction."

Patient takes a long breath. Pause. About fifteen seconds.

Clinician: "That was hard to hear."

Patient: "Yes. But I asked."

Values.

Clinician: "If your health situation worsens, what is most important to you?"

Patient: "I want to be home. I want to be with my husband. I do not want to die in a hospital."

Clinician: "Being home with your husband matters more than anything else."

Patient: "Yes."

Clinician: "What are you most worried about?"

Patient: "Pain. And being a burden on him."

Clinician: "You are worried about pain and about what he would have to do to care for you."

Patient: "Yes."

Clinician: "What gives you strength as you think about what is ahead?"

Patient: "My faith. And my husband. I have had a good life."

Recommendation.

Clinician: "You have told me that being home matters most, that you are worried about pain, that you do not want to be a burden, and that your faith and your husband carry you. Given those things, I would recommend we focus on hospice care at home, with a clear plan for pain management so you never have to be afraid of being in pain, and with enough support services that your husband is not doing this alone. Does that feel right to you?"

Patient: "Yes. That sounds right."

Clinician: "Is there anything about it that does not feel right, or that you would want to change?"

Patient: "No. That is what I want."

The whole conversation took about thirty five minutes. The resulting documentation would include direct quotes, the specific values named, and the plan agreed to. The next clinician who reads the note will know exactly what this patient wants and why.

Appendix D: MI Fidelity Self Assessment

This appendix adapts the Motivational Interviewing Treatment Integrity (MITI) coding framework for self assessment in end of life conversations. It is not a replacement for formal coding by a trained observer. It is a tool you can use on yourself, regularly, to notice patterns in your own practice.

D.1 Setup

Record one conversation per month. Use the MITI approach of scoring a twenty minute segment of conversation, not the whole visit. Get the patient's or family's written consent before recording. Many palliative care teams have consent templates. If yours does not, the basic language is: "I would like to record part of our conversation so I can review my own communication later. The recording will not go in your chart. It will only be used for my own learning. Is that okay with you?"

If recording is not feasible, do the self assessment from memory immediately after a visit, while details are fresh. Memory based assessment is less accurate than recording based but still useful.

D.2 Count Behaviors

In the twenty minute segment, count:

Open questions: Questions that invite broad answers and cannot be answered yes or no. Count each one.

Closed questions: Questions that can be answered yes, no, or with a number. Count each one.

Simple reflections: Statements that restate the speaker's words with slight modification, without adding meaning.

Complex reflections: Statements that add meaning, feeling, or implication the speaker did not explicitly state.

Affirmations: Specific, observable statements of the person's effort or strength. Generic praise ("you are doing great") does not count.

MI consistent behaviors: Seeking permission, emphasizing autonomy, supporting self direction.

MI inconsistent behaviors: Unsolicited advice or information without permission, warning, directing, confronting, moralizing, or using persuasion to press a point.

D.3 Calculate Summary Scores

From the behavior counts, calculate:

Reflection to question ratio: Total reflections divided by total questions. Target: at least 1:1. Proficient: 2:1 or higher.

Percent complex reflections: Complex reflections divided by total reflections, times 100. Target: at least 40 percent. Proficient: 50 percent or higher.

Percent open questions: Open questions divided by total questions, times 100. Target: majority open. Proficient: 70 percent or higher.

Percent MI consistent: MI consistent behaviors divided by (MI consistent + MI inconsistent) behaviors, times 100. Target: 90 percent or higher.

D.4 Rate Global Measures

On a scale of 1 (low) to 5 (high), rate yourself on each of the following:

Engagement: Did the conversation feel like a real connection, or like an interview? 1 = transactional, no rapport. 3 = some rapport, patient mostly answered questions. 5 = genuine connection, patient appeared to trust clinician.

Partnership: Did the patient feel like a collaborator, or like a recipient of care? 1 = clinician directed, patient passive. 3 = some collaboration, clinician still led. 5 = true partnership, patient's voice shaped the conversation.

Empathy: Did the clinician accurately understand and reflect the patient's experience? 1 = no reflection of patient experience. 3 = some reflection, missed major emotional content. 5 = deeply accurate reflection of patient's inner experience.

Autonomy support: Did the clinician emphasize the patient's right to make decisions? 1 = clinician directed decisions. 3 = some acknowledgment of patient choice. 5 = consistent emphasis on patient's autonomy.

Presence: Was the clinician present to the patient, or was the clinician watching the clock, managing the chart, or performing competence? 1 = clinician clearly distracted or performative. 3 = clinician mostly present, with some distraction. 5 = clinician fully with the patient.

D.5 Interpret Results

After the twenty minute segment:

If your reflection to question ratio is below 1:1, you are asking more than reflecting. Work on holding questions and reflecting instead.

If your percent complex reflections is below 40 percent, you are staying at the surface. Work on making complex guesses about what is underneath.

If your percent open questions is below 50 percent, you are using closed questions as your default. Work on opening with open questions.

If your percent MI consistent is below 90 percent, you are likely directing more than collaborating. Notice where you are giving advice without permission or pressing your point.

If any global score is below 3, that is a specific area for attention. Pick one to work on in the next month.

D.6 Track Over Time

Keep a simple log of your self assessments. Date, behavior counts, summary scores, global scores, and one sentence about what you want to work on next.

Over six months, you should see movement. Not dramatic. Small shifts. The reflection to question ratio creeping up. The percent complex reflections growing. One global score improving as you focus on it.

If you do not see movement after six months of attention, consider formal coaching or supervision. Your own eye on your own work has limits. Another trained eye can see what you cannot.

D.7 Worked Example

Recording of a twenty minute family meeting with a patient, wife, and daughter.

Behavior counts:

Open questions: 7 Closed questions: 4 Simple reflections: 5 Complex reflections: 8 Affirmations: 2 MI consistent: 3 MI inconsistent: 1

Summary scores:

Reflection to question ratio: 13 / 11 = 1.18. Meets target. Percent complex reflections: 8 / 13 = 62%. Proficient. Percent open questions: 7 / 11 = 64%. Below proficient, above target. Percent MI consistent: 3 / 4 = 75%. Below target.

Global scores:

Engagement: 4 Partnership: 3 Empathy: 4 Autonomy support: 3 Presence: 4

Interpretation: The ratio and complex reflection percentage are strong. The MI consistent score is below target, suggesting that the single MI inconsistent behavior was significant. On review of the recording, the clinician notices that they advised the family about hospice enrollment without first asking permission. That is the specific thing to work on next month. Partnership and autonomy support both scored 3, which is consistent with the finding that the clinician directed more than collaborated in this particular meeting.

Next month's focus: Ask permission before sharing information. Use elicit-provide-elicit more consistently.

Appendix E: Team Based Practice Exercises

These exercises are designed for interdisciplinary groups, typically 4 to 10 people, meeting for 30 to 90 minutes. They can be run by a designated facilitator or can rotate among team members. They are meant to be done repeatedly rather than once. Culture shifts through practice over time, not through single events.

E.1 Exercise One: The Reflection Round

Duration: 20 minutes. Group size: 4 to 8. Skill: Reflections, especially complex.

Setup: Everyone sits in a circle. The facilitator describes a single patient statement. Everyone writes down a reflection they would offer in response. Then each person shares their reflection, one at a time, around the circle.

Patient statement example: "I just don't know if I have the strength to keep doing this."

After each person shares their reflection, the group briefly notes if it was simple (restatement) or complex (added meaning), and if it named feeling, value, or implication.

After the full round, the facilitator offers a new statement and repeats.

Variations: Use real statements the team has heard recently (anonymized). Rotate who proposes the patient statement.

What this builds: The habit of generating reflections, and the ear for the difference between simple and complex.

E.2 Exercise Two: The Two Minute Role Play

Duration: 30 to 45 minutes total; 2 minutes per round. Group size: 3 to 6. Skill: Single MI move applied in real time.

Setup: Pair up. One person plays the patient or family member. The other plays the clinician. The facilitator announces the scenario (e.g., "a caregiver who is refusing to give morphine") and the skill focus (e.g., "complex reflections only, no questions").

The clinician has two minutes to demonstrate the target skill. The patient plays the scenario.

Debrief: After each two minute round, the pair spends two minutes talking about what worked and what was hard. Then switch roles.

Run three to five rounds with different scenarios and different skill focuses.

What this builds: Comfort with specific MI moves under light pressure. The two minute constraint prevents overthinking.

E.3 Exercise Three: The Anonymized Recording Review

Duration: 45 to 60 minutes. Group size: 4 to 10. Skill: Identifying MI moves, listening for missed opportunities.

Setup: One team member volunteers a short recording (with patient consent) of a conversation they led. Five to ten minutes is usually enough. Names are removed or changed.

The group listens to the recording together. After each significant exchange, the facilitator pauses the recording and asks: "What did you notice? What did the clinician do well? What was a missed opportunity?"

After the full recording, the facilitator invites the clinician whose recording it is to reflect: "What did you learn from hearing your own work?"

Ground rules: Critique the work, not the person. Feedback is specific and constructive. The volunteer has the right to end the exercise at any time.

What this builds: A shared language for discussing communication craft. Willingness to be observed and to observe others.

E.4 Exercise Four: The Elephant Exercise

Duration: 30 to 45 minutes. Group size: 4 to 8. Skill: Naming unspoken dynamics in family meetings.

Setup: The facilitator describes a family scenario with an unspoken elephant. For example: "Family of three adult siblings meeting about their father's care. The oldest has been absent for years and flew in yesterday. The other two have been caring for him. The elephant is that the other two resent the oldest, but nobody will say so."

The group discusses: how would you name this elephant? What language would you use? What is the risk of naming it? What is the risk of not naming it?

After discussion, one person demonstrates a naming attempt in the room, with others playing the family members. The group gives feedback.

Run two to three scenarios.

What this builds: Willingness to name what is visible. Calibration of tone and timing.

E.5 Exercise Five: The Permission Practice

Duration: 20 minutes. Group size: 4 to 6. Skill: Seeking permission before sharing information or advice.

Setup: Pair up. One person plays a patient or family member who is asking for information. The other plays the clinician. The clinician's constraint: they cannot share any information until they have sought permission in a specific, non formulaic way.

Patient example: "What do you think is going to happen to my mother in the next few weeks?"

The clinician has to ask permission before answering. Bad permission seeking: "Can I share what I am thinking?" (too generic). Good permission seeking: "I can share what I am seeing in her current condition and what that often looks like over time. Is that helpful, or would you rather we talk about something else first?"

Run three to five rounds.

What this builds: Specific, non formulaic permission seeking. Awareness of when advice is being given without invitation.

E.6 Exercise Six: The Difficult Debrief

Duration: 60 to 90 minutes. Group size: 4 to 8. Skill: Reflective practice on hard cases.

Setup: One team member presents a recent case that was hard for them personally. Not a case review. A personal reflection. The structure: what happened, what was hard, what they carried out of it, what they wish they had done differently, what they are still sitting with.

The group's role: listen without fixing. No problem solving. After the presentation, group members reflect back what they heard. They may share briefly what the case brought up in them, if it did.

Ground rules: No advice. No suggestions for what to do differently next time. The purpose is to witness the experience, not to coach.

The facilitator closes by asking the presenter: "What are you taking from this conversation?"

What this builds: A team culture in which the work of the work can be discussed without performance. Reduces cumulative grief through shared processing.

E.7 Exercise Seven: The Goals Of Care Rehearsal

Duration: 45 minutes. Group size: 4 to 6. Skill: Full goals of care conversation, start to finish.

Setup: One person plays a patient with a defined clinical scenario (e.g., 78 year old with metastatic lung cancer, six months since diagnosis, two lines of treatment, now progressing). Another plays the clinician. A third acts as observer.

The clinician has fifteen minutes to run a goals of care conversation, aiming to reach a specific values based plan by the end.

After fifteen minutes, the observer provides feedback using a structured framework: what did the clinician do that worked, what was missed, what was a specific recommendation for next time.

Then switch roles and run a second round with a different scenario.

What this builds: Integrated practice of multiple MI skills in a longer conversation. Ability to move through the four phases of engaging, focusing, evoking, and planning.

E.8 Facilitator Notes

For any of these exercises:

Start with psychological safety. The first exercise you run should be low stakes. Do not start with the Difficult Debrief.

Rotate who leads. Facilitator skill grows through practice. Distribute the role.

Keep it regular. A single exercise is an event. A regular practice (every two weeks, every month) is a culture.

Follow up outside the exercise. The moves practiced in the exercise need to show up in real work. Individual supervision or peer coaching supports this transfer.

Protect confidentiality. Recordings, case details, and personal reflections shared in the group stay in the group.

Celebrate visibly. When a team member tries something from an exercise and it works in real practice, name it in rounds. "Gemma used a complex reflection in the Patel family meeting yesterday that shifted the conversation. I want to name that." This reinforces the practice.

Appendix F: Reproducible Handouts For Families

This appendix contains four handouts that can be printed and given to families. Each is one page or less. The language is deliberately plain. Photocopy permission is granted for clinical use.

F.1 Handout One: What To Expect In The Last Days

When someone is in the last days of life, their body changes in specific ways. These changes are normal. Knowing what to expect can help you feel more prepared and less afraid.

Breathing changes. Breathing may become slower, faster, or uneven. There may be pauses between breaths. This is normal. It is the body's work.

Less interest in food and water. Your loved one may stop wanting to eat or drink. The body needs less as it slows down. Forcing food can cause discomfort. Small sips of water or ice chips can help with dry mouth. Moistening the lips with a swab is usually more helpful than giving fluids.

Sleeping more. Your loved one may sleep most of the day. They may be harder to wake. This is the body conserving energy.

Restlessness. Sometimes, a person near the end of life becomes restless. They may pick at the blankets or seem agitated. Medications can help. Tell the nurse if this happens.

Changes in skin color. Hands, feet, and knees may become cool, pale, or blotchy. This is because circulation is slowing.

Sounds when breathing. There may be a rattling or gurgling sound with breathing. This is fluid in the throat. It is usually not uncomfortable for the person. Gently turning their head to the side can help.

Withdrawal. Your loved one may seem less responsive to people and the room. This is normal. They may still hear you. Talking to them, playing their favorite music, or holding their hand can all be comforting.

When death comes. There is usually a last breath, followed by no more breathing. This may be peaceful. Take the time you need. There is no rush. Call the hospice team when you are ready.

If you have any questions or concerns, call the hospice line. Someone is available 24 hours a day.

F.2 Handout Two: How To Be With Someone Who Is Dying

Many people do not know what to do when they are with someone who is dying. Here are some things that often help.

Be there. Just your presence matters. You do not have to say anything.

Talk to them. Even if your loved one seems not to hear, they may still be able to. Share memories. Tell them you love them. Say the things you want to say.

Touch. Hold their hand. Stroke their forehead. Touch is one of the last senses to fade.

Play their favorite music. Songs from earlier in life often reach people who do not respond to much else.

Read to them. A favorite book, scripture, or poetry.

Let them sleep. Waking them is not necessary. Your being there matters even if they are asleep.

Keep the room quiet and soft. Low lights. Soft voices. Minimal clatter.

Take care of yourself. You cannot sit at the bedside around the clock. Take breaks. Eat. Sleep. Let other family members take turns.

Say what you want to say. If there is something you have wanted to tell them, say it now. Even if they cannot respond, speaking the words matters.

Be patient with yourself. You may cry. You may laugh. You may not know what you feel. All of it is okay.

If you need support, the hospice team is available. Chaplains, social workers, and nurses can all be called.

F.3 Handout Three: After The Death

When your loved one dies, you do not need to rush. Take your time.

Right after the death. There is no need to call anyone immediately. Sit with your loved one as long as you want. This may be a few minutes or many hours. There is no wrong choice.

Calling the hospice. When you are ready, call the hospice line. The on call nurse will come to the home to confirm the death and help you with next steps.

The body. The nurse will help you decide when to call the funeral home. You can ask the funeral home to come right away or to wait a few hours. Many families find that having time with the body, before it is taken, is important to them.

Other people who need to know. The hospice nurse can help you think about who to call and when. There is no requirement to call everyone immediately.

Medications and equipment. The hospice will pick up any unused medications and equipment after the death. You do not need to worry about this right away.

Paperwork. A death certificate will be filed. The funeral home usually coordinates this. You will receive copies.

In the weeks that follow. The hospice team will contact you about bereavement support. You will receive information about support groups and counseling if you want them.

Grief. Grief comes in waves. Some days are harder than others. Anniversaries and holidays can be particularly hard. There is no timeline for grief. Be gentle with the pace you need.

When to reach out for help. If you are having trouble sleeping or eating, if you are feeling hopeless, if you cannot function for weeks at a time, please reach out. The hospice bereavement team can help. So can your own doctor. Grief is natural. Grief that is interfering with your life is something to get help with.

F.4 Handout Four: Questions To Ask Your Care Team

You may feel there are things you want to know but do not know how to ask. Here are some questions many families find helpful.

About the illness:

What is happening now in his body?

What changes might we see in the next few days or weeks?

Is she in pain? How would we know?

What would be a sign that things are getting worse quickly?

About care:

What medications is she on, and what is each one for?

Is there anything we can do that would help her be more comfortable?

What should we do if she has a new symptom, like trouble breathing?

Who should we call, and when?

About what to expect:

What are the signs that death is near?

What will the last hours look like?

Will she be in pain at the end?

Can we be with her when it happens?

About ourselves:

How can we take care of ourselves while we are caring for her?

Is there someone we can talk to about what we are feeling?

What help is available if we need a break?

What can we do for our children, who are also hurting?

About after:

What do we need to do when the death happens?

How long can we stay with her after she dies?

Who do we call, and when?

What happens next?

About grief:

Is there a support group we can join?

Is counseling available?

What if we need help in the weeks or months after?

You can write down questions as they come to you. Bring them to the next visit. There is no wrong question. You deserve to know what is happening.

References

- Abbott, K. H., Sago, J. G., Breen, C. M., Abernethy, A. P., & Tulsky, J. A. (2001). Families looking back: One year after discussion of withdrawal or withholding of life-sustaining support. *Critical Care Medicine, 29*(1), 197–201.
- Ariadne Labs. (n.d.). *Serious illness care.*
- American Academy of Pediatrics, Committee on Hospital Care, & Institute for Patient- and Family-Centered Care. (2012). Patient- and family-centered care and the pediatrician's role. *Pediatrics, 129*(2), 394–404.
- Apodaca, T. R., & Longabaugh, R. (2009). Mechanisms of change in motivational interviewing: A review and preliminary evaluation of the evidence. *Addiction, 104*(5), 705–715.
- Apodaca, T. R., Jackson, K. M., Borsari, B., Magill, M., Longabaugh, R., Mastroleo, N. R., & Barnett, N. P. (2016). Which individual therapist behaviors elicit client change talk and sustain talk in motivational interviewing? *Journal of Substance Abuse Treatment, 61*, 60–65.
- Arnold, R. M., Back, A. L., Baile, W. F., Edwards, K. A., & Tulsky, J. A. (2010). The Oncotalk/VitalTalk model. In R. A. Kissane, D. W. Bultz, P. N. Butow, C. L. Bylund, S. Noble, & S. Wilkinson (Eds.), *Handbook of communication in oncology and palliative care.* Oxford University Press.
- Azoulay, E., Timsit, J.-F., Sprung, C. L., Soares, M., Rusinova, K., Lafabrie, A., Abizanda, R., Svantesson, M., Rubulotta, F., Ricou, B., Benoit, D., Heyland, D., Joynt, G., Français, A., Azevedo Maia, P., Owczuk, R., Benbenishty, J., de Vita, M., Valentin, A., ... Schlemmer, B. (2009). Prevalence and factors of intensive care unit conflicts: The Conflicus study. *American Journal of Respiratory and Critical Care Medicine, 180*(9), 853–860.
- Back, A. L., Arnold, R. M., & Quill, T. E. (2003). Hope for the best, and prepare for the worst. *Annals of Internal Medicine, 138*(5), 439–443.

- Back, A. L., Arnold, R. M., & Tulsky, J. A. (2009). *Mastering communication with seriously ill patients: Balancing honesty with empathy and hope*. Cambridge University Press.
- Back, A. L., Arnold, R. M., Baile, W. F., Fryer-Edwards, K. A., Alexander, S. C., Barley, G. E., Gooley, T. A., & Tulsky, J. A. (2007). Efficacy of communication skills training for giving bad news and discussing transitions to palliative care. *Archives of Internal Medicine, 167*(5), 453–460.
- Back, A. L., Arnold, R. M., Baile, W. F., Tulsky, J. A., & Fryer-Edwards, K. (2005). Approaching difficult communication tasks in oncology. *CA: A Cancer Journal for Clinicians, 55*(3), 164–177.
- Baile, W. F., Buckman, R., Lenzi, R., Glober, G., Beale, E. A., & Kudelka, A. P. (2000). SPIKES—A six-step protocol for delivering bad news: Application to the patient with cancer. *The Oncologist, 5*(4), 302–311.
- Bakitas, M., Lyons, K. D., Hegel, M. T., Balan, S., Brokaw, F. C., Seville, J., Hull, J. G., Li, Z., Tosteson, T. D., Byock, I. R., & Ahles, T. A. (2009). Effects of a palliative care intervention on clinical outcomes in patients with advanced cancer. *JAMA, 302*(7), 741–749.
- Balboni, T. A., Paulk, M. E., Balboni, M. J., Phelps, A. C., Loggers, E. T., Wright, A. A., Block, S. D., Lewis, E. F., Peteet, J. R., & Prigerson, H. G. (2010). Provision of spiritual care to patients with advanced cancer: Associations with medical care and quality of life near death. *Journal of Clinical Oncology, 28*(3), 445–452.
- Beckman, H. B., & Frankel, R. M. (1984). The effect of physician behavior on the collection of data. *Annals of Internal Medicine, 101*(5), 692–696.
- Berger, J. T. (1998). Culture and ethnicity in clinical care. *Archives of Internal Medicine, 158*(19), 2085–2090.
- Bernacki, R. E., & Block, S. D. (2014). Communication about serious illness care goals: A review and synthesis of best practices. *JAMA Internal Medicine, 174*(12), 1994–2003.

- Bernacki, R., Paladino, J., Neville, B. A., Hutchings, M., Kavanagh, J., Geerse, O. P., Lakin, J., Sanders, J. J., Miller, K., Lipsitz, S., Gawande, A. A., & Block, S. D. (2019). Effect of the Serious Illness Care Program in outpatient oncology: A cluster randomized clinical trial. *JAMA Internal Medicine, 179*(6), 751–759.
- Billings, J. A. (2011). The end-of-life family meeting in intensive care, part I: Indications, outcomes, and family needs. *Journal of Palliative Medicine, 14*(9), 1042–1050.
- Black, I., & Helgason, A. R. (2018). Using motivational interviewing to facilitate death talk in end-of-life care: An ethical analysis. *BMC Palliative Care, 17*(1), Article 51.
- Blackhall, L. J., Murphy, S. T., Frank, G., Michel, V., & Azen, S. (1995). Ethnicity and attitudes toward patient autonomy. *JAMA, 274*(10), 820–825.
- Butler, R. N. (1963). The life review: An interpretation of reminiscence in the aged. *Psychiatry, 26*(1), 65–76.
- Carson, S. S., Cox, C. E., Wallenstein, S., Hanson, L. C., Danis, M., Tulsky, J. A., Chai, E., & Nelson, J. E. (2016). Effect of palliative care-led meetings for families of patients with chronic critical illness: A randomized clinical trial. *JAMA, 316*(1), 51–62.
- Casarett, D. J., & Quill, T. E. (2007). "I'm not ready for hospice": Strategies for timely and effective hospice discussions. *Annals of Internal Medicine, 146*(6), 443–449.
- Casarett, D., Crowley, R., Stevenson, C., Xie, S., & Teno, J. (2005). Making difficult decisions about hospice enrollment: What do patients and families want to know? *Journal of the American Geriatrics Society, 53*(2), 249–254.
- Casarett, D., Kapo, J., & Caplan, A. (2005). Appropriate use of artificial nutrition and hydration: Fundamental principles and recommendations. *New England Journal of Medicine, 353*(24), 2607–2612.
- Childers, J. W., Back, A. L., Tulsky, J. A., & Arnold, R. M. (2017). REMAP: A framework for goals-of-care conversations. *Journal of Oncology Practice, 13*(10), e844–e850.

- Chochinov, H. M., Hack, T., Hassard, T., Kristjanson, L. J., McClement, S., & Harlos, M. (2005). Dignity therapy: A novel psychotherapeutic intervention for patients near the end of life. *Journal of Clinical Oncology, 23*(24), 5520–5525.
- Christakis, N. A. (1999). *Death foretold: Prophecy and prognosis in medical care*. University of Chicago Press.
- Christakis, N. A., & Lamont, E. B. (2000). Extent and determinants of error in doctors' prognoses in terminally ill patients: Prospective cohort study. *BMJ, 320*(7233), 469–473.
- Cohen-Mansfield, J., Werner, P., & Reisberg, B. (1995). Temporal order of cognitive and functional loss in a nursing home population. *Journal of the American Geriatrics Society, 43*(9), 974–978.
- Committee on Bioethics. (2016). Informed consent in decision-making in pediatric practice. *Pediatrics, 138*(2), e20161484.
- Connor, S. R., Pyenson, B., Fitch, K., Spence, C., & Iwasaki, K. (2007). Comparing hospice and nonhospice patient survival among patients who die within a three-year window. *Journal of Pain and Symptom Management, 33*(3), 238–246.
- Crawley, L. M., Marshall, P. A., Lo, B., & Koenig, B. A. (2002). Strategies for culturally effective end-of-life care. *Annals of Internal Medicine, 136*(9), 673–679.
- Curtis, J. R., Back, A. L., Ford, D. W., Downey, L., Shannon, S. E., Doorenbos, A. Z., Kross, E. K., Reinke, L. F., Feemster, L. C., Edlund, B., Arnold, R. W., O'Connor, K., & Engelberg, R. A. (2013). Effect of communication skills training for residents and nurse practitioners on quality of communication with patients with serious illness. *JAMA, 310*(21), 2271–2281.
- Curtis, J. R., Treece, P. D., Nielsen, E. L., Gold, J., Ciechanowski, P. S., Shannon, S. E., Khandelwal, N., Young, J. P., & Engelberg, R. A. (2016). Randomized trial of communication facilitators to reduce family distress and intensity of end-of-life care. *American Journal of Respiratory and Critical Care Medicine, 193*(2), 154–162.

- Damschroder, L. J., Aron, D. C., Keith, R. E., Kirsh, S. R., Alexander, J. A., & Lowery, J. C. (2009). Fostering implementation of health services research findings into practice: A consolidated framework for advancing implementation science. *Implementation Science, 4*, Article 50.
- Detering, K. M., Hancock, A. D., Reade, M. C., & Silvester, W. (2010). The impact of advance care planning on end-of-life care in elderly patients: Randomised controlled trial. *BMJ, 340*, c1345.
- Emanuel, L. L., Ferris, F. D., von Gunten, C. F., & Von Roenn, J. (2011). *The last hours of living: Practical advice for clinicians*. Medscape.
- Enzinger, A. C., Zhang, B., Schrag, D., & Prigerson, H. G. (2015). Outcomes of prognostic disclosure: Associations with prognostic understanding, distress, and relationship with physician among patients with advanced cancer. *Journal of Clinical Oncology, 33*(32), 3809–3816.
- Epstein, R. M., & Street, R. L. (2007). *Patient-centered communication in cancer care: Promoting healing and reducing suffering*. National Cancer Institute.
- Epstein, R. M., & Street, R. L. (2011). Shared mind: Communication, decision making, and autonomy in serious illness. *Annals of Family Medicine, 9*(5), 454–461.
- Ferrell, B. R., Temel, J. S., Temin, S., Alesi, E. R., Balboni, T. A., Basch, E. M., Firn, J. I., Paice, J. A., Peppercorn, J. M., Phillips, T., Stovall, E. L., Zimmermann, C., & Smith, T. J. (2017). Integration of palliative care into standard oncology care: American Society of Clinical Oncology clinical practice guideline update. *Journal of Clinical Oncology, 35*(1), 96–112.
- Feudtner, C., Friebert, S., & Jewell, J. (2013). Pediatric palliative care and hospice care commitments, guidelines, and recommendations. *Pediatrics, 132*(5), 966–972.
- Figley, C. R. (2002). Compassion fatigue: Psychotherapists' chronic lack of self-care. *Journal of Clinical Psychology, 58*(11), 1433–1441.

- Finucane, T. E., Christmas, C., & Travis, K. (1999). Tube feeding in patients with advanced dementia: A review of the evidence. *JAMA, 282*(14), 1365–1370.
- Flores, G. (2005). The impact of medical interpreter services on the quality of health care: A systematic review. *Medical Care Research and Review, 62*(3), 255–299.
- Forsetlund, L., O'Brien, M. A., Forsén, L., Reinar, L. M., Okwen, M. P., Horsley, T., & Rose, C. J. (2021). Continuing education meetings and workshops: Effects on professional practice and healthcare outcomes. *Cochrane Database of Systematic Reviews, 2021*(9), CD003030.
- Fromme, E. K., Zive, D., Schmidt, T. A., Olszewski, E., & Tolle, S. W. (2012). POLST Registry do-not-resuscitate orders and other patient treatment preferences. *JAMA, 307*(1), 34–35.
- Gawande, A. (2014). *Being mortal: Medicine and what matters in the end.* Metropolitan Books.
- Glajchen, M., Goehring, A., Johns, H., & Portenoy, R. K. (2022). Family meetings in palliative care: Benefits and barriers. *Current Treatment Options in Oncology, 23*(5), 658–667.
- Glare, P., Virik, K., Jones, M., Hudson, M., Eychmuller, S., Simes, J., & Christakis, N. (2003). A systematic review of physicians' survival predictions in terminally ill cancer patients. *BMJ, 327*(7408), 195–198.
- Goldberg, R. J. (1984). Disclosure of information to adult cancer patients: Issues and update. *Journal of Clinical Oncology, 2*(8), 948–955.
- Halifax, J. (2008). *Being with dying: Cultivating compassion and fearlessness in the presence of death.* Shambhala.
- Harrison, R. L., & Westwood, M. J. (2009). Preventing vicarious traumatization of mental health therapists: Identifying protective practices. *Psychotherapy, 46*(2), 203–219.
- Heuberger, R. A. (2010). Artificial nutrition and hydration at the end of life. *Journal of Nutrition for the Elderly, 29*(4), 347–385.

- Heyland, D. K., Barwich, D., Pichora, D., Dodek, P., Lamontagne, F., You, J., Taylor, C., Porterfield, P., Sinuff, T., & Simon, J. (2013). Failure to engage hospitalized elderly patients and their families in advance care planning. *JAMA Internal Medicine, 173*(9), 778–787.
- Heyland, D. K., Cook, D. J., Rocker, G. M., Dodek, P. M., Kutsogiannis, D. J., Skrobik, Y., Jiang, X., Day, A. G., & Cohen, S. R. (2010). Defining priorities for improving end-of-life care in Canada. *Canadian Medical Association Journal, 182*(16), E747–E752.
- Hinds, P. S., Oakes, L. L., Hicks, J., Powell, B., Srivastava, D. K., Spunt, S. L., Harper, J., Baker, J. N., West, N. K., & Furman, W. L. (2009). "Trying to be a good parent" as defined by interviews with parents who made phase I, terminal care, and resuscitation decisions for their children. *Journal of Clinical Oncology, 27*(35), 5979–5985.
- Houck, J. M., & Moyers, T. B. (2015). Within-session communication patterns predict alcohol treatment outcomes. *Drug and Alcohol Dependence, 157*, 205–209.
- Hudson, P., Thomas, T., Quinn, K., & Aranda, S. (2009). Family meetings in palliative care: Are they effective? *Palliative Medicine, 23*(2), 150–157.
- Jacobsen, J., Alexander-Scott, N., Blinderman, C., Jackson, V., & Meier, D. E. (2018). "I'd recommend ..." How to incorporate your recommendation into shared decision making for patients with serious illness. *Journal of Pain and Symptom Management, 55*(4), 1224–1230.
- Jacobsen, J., Brenner, K., Greer, J. A., Jacobo, M., Rosenberg, L., Nipp, R. D., & Jackson, V. A. (2018). When a patient is reluctant to talk about it: A dual framework to focus on living well and tolerate the possibility of dying. *Journal of Palliative Medicine, 21*(3), 322–327.
- Jansen, J., van Weert, J. C. M., de Groot, J., van Dulmen, S., Heeren, T. J., & Bensing, J. M. (2008). Emotional and informational patient cues: The impact of nurses' responses on recall. *Patient Education and Counseling, 72*(2), 252–260.
- Jansen, L. A., & Sulmasy, D. P. (2002). Sedation, alimentation, hydration, and equivocation: Careful

conversation about care at the end of life. *Annals of Internal Medicine, 136*(11), 845–849.

- Kagawa-Singer, M., & Blackhall, L. J. (2001). Negotiating cross-cultural issues at the end of life: "You got to go where he lives." *JAMA, 286*(23), 2993–3001.
- Kaldjian, L. C., Curtis, A. E., Shinkunas, L. A., & Cannon, K. T. (2008). Goals of care toward the end of life: A structured literature review. *American Journal of Hospice and Palliative Medicine, 25*(6), 501–511.
- Kearney, M. K., Weininger, R. B., Vachon, M. L. S., Harrison, R. L., & Mount, B. M. (2009). Self-care of physicians caring for patients at the end of life: "Being connected ... a key to my survival." *JAMA, 301*(11), 1155–1164.
- Kissane, D. W., & Bloch, S. (2002). *Family-focused grief therapy: A model of family-centered care during palliative care and bereavement.* Open University Press.
- Kissane, D. W., & Parnes, F. (2014). *Bereavement care for families.* Routledge.
- Ko, E., Kwak, J., & Nelson-Becker, H. (2015). What constitutes a good and bad death? Perspectives of homeless older adults. *Death Studies, 39*(7), 422–432.
- Kolanowski, A., Mogle, J., Fick, D. M., Hill, N., Mulhall, P., Nadler, J., Colancecco, E., & Behrens, L. (2011). Preliminary cognitive impairment predictors of delirium severity in hospitalized elderly persons with dementia. *Research in Gerontological Nursing, 4*(1), 26–35.
- Kramer, B. J., Boelk, A. Z., & Auer, C. (2006). Family conflict at the end of life: Lessons learned in a model program for vulnerable older adults. *Journal of Palliative Medicine, 9*(3), 791–801.
- Kramer, B. J., Kavanaugh, M., Trentham-Dietz, A., Walsh, M., & Yonker, J. A. (2010). Predictors of family conflict at the end of life: The experience of spouses and adult children of persons with lung cancer. *The Gerontologist, 50*(2), 215–225.
- Kreicbergs, U., Valdimarsdottir, U., Onelov, E., Henter, J.-I., & Steineck, G. (2004). Talking about death with children

who have severe malignant disease. *New England Journal of Medicine, 351*(12), 1175–1186.

- Kwon, J. H. (2014). Overcoming barriers in cancer pain management. *Journal of Clinical Oncology, 32*(16), 1727–1733.
- Lamont, E. B., & Christakis, N. A. (2001). Prognostic disclosure to patients with cancer near the end of life. *Annals of Internal Medicine, 134*(12), 1096–1105.
- Lautrette, A., Darmon, M., Megarbane, B., Joly, L.-M., Chevret, S., Adrie, C., Barnoud, D., Bleichner, G., Bruel, C., Choukroun, G., Curtis, J. R., Fieux, F., Galliot, R., Garrouste-Orgeas, M., Georges, H., Goldgran-Toledano, D., Jourdain, M., Loubert, G., Reignier, J., ... Azoulay, E. (2007). A communication strategy and brochure for relatives of patients dying in the ICU. *New England Journal of Medicine, 356*(5), 469–478.
- Lopez, V., Copp, G., & Molassiotis, A. (2012). Male caregivers of patients with breast and gynecologic cancer. *Cancer Nursing, 35*(6), 431–440.
- Lorig, K. R., Sobel, D. S., Ritter, P. L., Laurent, D., & Hobbs, M. (2001). Effect of a self-management program on patients with chronic disease. *Effective Clinical Practice, 4*(6), 256–262.
- Mack, J. W., Weeks, J. C., Wright, A. A., Block, S. D., & Prigerson, H. G. (2010). End-of-life discussions, goal attainment, and distress at the end of life: Predictors and outcomes of receipt of care consistent with preferences. *Journal of Clinical Oncology, 28*(7), 1203–1208.
- Mack, J. W., Wolfe, J., Grier, H. E., Cleary, P. D., & Weeks, J. C. (2006). Communication about prognosis between parents and physicians of children with cancer: Parent preferences and the impact of prognostic information. *Journal of Clinical Oncology, 24*(33), 5265–5270.
- Magill, M., Apodaca, T. R., Borsari, B., Gaume, J., Hoadley, A., Gordon, R. E. F., Tonigan, J. S., & Moyers, T. (2018). A meta-analysis of motivational interviewing process: Technical, relational, and conditional process

models of change. *Journal of Consulting and Clinical Psychology, 86*(2), 140–157.

- Marvel, M. K., Epstein, R. M., Flowers, K., & Beckman, H. B. (1999). Soliciting the patient's agenda: Have we improved? *JAMA, 281*(3), 283–287.
- Maslach, C., & Leiter, M. P. (2016). Understanding the burnout experience: Recent research and its implications for psychiatry. *World Psychiatry, 15*(2), 103–111.
- Meier, D. E., Ahronheim, J. C., Morris, J., Baskin-Lyons, S., & Morrison, R. S. (2001). High short-term mortality in hospitalized patients with advanced dementia: Lack of benefit of tube feeding. *Archives of Internal Medicine, 161*(4), 594–599.
- Miller, W. R., & Rollnick, S. (2023). *Motivational interviewing: Helping people change and grow* (4th ed.). Guilford Press.
- Miller, W. R., & Rose, G. S. (2015). Motivational interviewing and decisional balance: Contrasting responses to client ambivalence. *Behavioural and Cognitive Psychotherapy, 43*(2), 129–141.
- Mitchell, S. L., Teno, J. M., Kiely, D. K., Shaffer, M. L., Jones, R. N., Prigerson, H. G., Volicer, L., Givens, J. L., & Hamel, M. B. (2009). The clinical course of advanced dementia. *New England Journal of Medicine, 361*(16), 1529–1538.
- Moore, P. M., Rivera, S., Bravo-Soto, G. A., Olivares, C., & Lawrie, T. A. (2018). Communication skills training for healthcare professionals working with people who have cancer. *Cochrane Database of Systematic Reviews, 2018*(7), CD003751.
- Morse, D. S., Edwardsen, E. A., & Gordon, H. S. (2008). Missed opportunities for interval empathy in lung cancer communication. *Archives of Internal Medicine, 168*(17), 1853–1858.
- Moyers, T. B., Rowell, L. N., Manuel, J. K., Ernst, D., & Houck, J. M. (2016). The Motivational Interviewing Treatment Integrity Code (MITI 4): Rationale, preliminary reliability and validity. *Journal of Substance Abuse Treatment, 65*, 36–42.

- Northouse, L. L., Katapodi, M. C., Song, L., Zhang, L., & Mood, D. W. (2010). Interventions with family caregivers of cancer patients: Meta-analysis of randomized trials. *CA: A Cancer Journal for Clinicians, 60*(5), 317–339.
- Nouwen, H. J. M., McNeill, D. P., & Morrison, D. A. (1982). *Compassion: A reflection on the Christian life*. Doubleday.
- Ogrinc, G., Davies, L., Goodman, D., Batalden, P., Davidoff, F., & Stevens, D. (2016). SQUIRE 2.0 (Standards for QUality Improvement Reporting Excellence): Revised publication guidelines from a detailed consensus process. *BMJ Quality & Safety, 25*(12), 986–992.
- Paladino, J., Bernacki, R., Neville, B. A., Kavanagh, J., Miranda, S. P., Palmor, M., Lakin, J., Desai, M., Lamas, D., Sanders, J. J., Gass, J., Henrich, N., Lipsitz, S., Fromme, E., Gawande, A. A., & Block, S. D. (2019). Evaluating an intervention to improve communication between oncology clinicians and patients with life-limiting cancer. *JAMA Oncology, 5*(6), 801–809.
- Paladino, J., Lakin, J. R., & Sanders, J. J. (2019). Communication strategies for sharing prognostic information with patients: Beyond survival statistics. *JAMA, 322*(14), 1345–1346.
- Palecek, E. J., Teno, J. M., Casarett, D. J., Hanson, L. C., Rhodes, R. L., & Mitchell, S. L. (2010). Comfort feeding only: A proposal to bring clarity to decision making regarding difficulty with eating for persons with advanced dementia. *Journal of the American Geriatrics Society, 58*(3), 580–584.
- Pereira, S. M., Fonseca, A. M., & Carvalho, A. S. (2011). Burnout in palliative care: A systematic review. *Nursing Ethics, 18*(3), 317–326.
- Periyakoil, V. S., Neri, E., & Kraemer, H. (2015). No easy talk: A mixed-methods study of doctor-reported barriers to conducting effective end-of-life conversations with diverse patients. *PLOS ONE, 10*(4), e0122321.
- Phelps, A. C., Maciejewski, P. K., Nilsson, M., Balboni, T. A., Wright, A. A., Paulk, M. E., Trice, E., Schrag, D.,

Peteet, J. R., Block, S. D., & Prigerson, H. G. (2009). Religious coping and use of intensive life-prolonging care near death in patients with advanced cancer. *JAMA, 301*(11), 1140–1147.

- Pollak, K. I., Alexander, S. C., Tulsky, J. A., Lyna, P., Coffman, C. J., Dolor, R. J., Gulbrandsen, P., & Østbye, T. (2011). Physician empathy and listening: Associations with patient satisfaction and autonomy. *Journal of the American Board of Family Medicine, 24*(6), 665–672.
- Pollak, K. I., Arnold, R. M., Jeffreys, A. S., Alexander, S. C., Olsen, M. K., Abernethy, A. P., Sugg Skinner, C., Rodriguez, K. L., & Tulsky, J. A. (2007). Oncologist communication about emotion during visits with patients with advanced cancer. *Journal of Clinical Oncology, 25*(36), 5748–5752.
- Pollak, K. I., Childers, J. W., & Arnold, R. M. (2011). Applying motivational interviewing techniques to palliative care communication. *Journal of Palliative Medicine, 14*(5), 587–592.
- Pollak, K. I., Jones, J., Lum, H. D., De La Cruz, S., Felton, S., Gill, A., & Kutner, J. S. (2015). Patient and caregiver opinions of motivational interviewing techniques in role-played palliative care conversations: A pilot study. *Journal of Pain and Symptom Management, 50*(1), 91–98.
- Portenoy, R. K., Sibirceva, U., Smout, R., Horn, S., Connor, S., Blum, R. H., Spence, C., & Fine, P. G. (2006). Opioid use and survival at the end of life: A survey of a hospice population. *Journal of Pain and Symptom Management, 32*(6), 532–540.
- Puchalski, C. M. (2006). Spiritual assessment in clinical practice. *Psychiatric Annals, 36*(3), 150–155.
- Quill, T. E. (2000). Perspectives on care at the close of life. Initiating end-of-life discussions with seriously ill patients: Addressing the elephant in the room. *JAMA, 284*(19), 2502–2507.
- Quill, T. E., & Brody, H. (1996). Physician recommendations and patient autonomy: Finding a balance between physician power and patient choice. *Annals of Internal Medicine, 125*(9), 763–769.

- Quill, T. E., Arnold, R., & Back, A. L. (2009). Discussing treatment preferences with patients who want "everything." *Annals of Internal Medicine, 151*(5), 345–349.
- Quill, T. E., Dresser, R., & Brock, D. W. (1997). The rule of double effect: A critique of its role in end-of-life decision making. *New England Journal of Medicine, 337*(24), 1768–1771.
- Raijmakers, N. J. H., van Zuylen, L., Costantini, M., Caraceni, A., Clark, J., Lundquist, G., Voltz, R., Ellershaw, J. E., & van der Heide, A. (2011). Artificial nutrition and hydration in the last week of life in cancer patients: A systematic literature review of practices and effects. *Annals of Oncology, 22*(7), 1478–1486.
- Reisberg, B. (1988). Functional assessment staging (FAST). *Psychopharmacology Bulletin, 24*(4), 653–659.
- Reisfield, G. M., & Wilson, G. R. (2007). Rational use of sublingual opioids in palliative medicine. *Journal of Palliative Medicine, 10*(2), 465–475.
- Remen, R. N. (1996). *Kitchen table wisdom: Stories that heal*. Riverhead Books.
- Rollnick, S., Miller, W. R., & Butler, C. C. (2022). *Motivational interviewing in health care: Helping patients change behavior* (2nd ed.). Guilford Press.
- Rosenberg, A. R., Starks, H., Unguru, Y., Feudtner, C., & Diekema, D. (2017). Truth telling in the setting of cultural differences and incurable pediatric illness. *JAMA Pediatrics, 171*(11), 1113–1119.
- Rosenberg, A. R., Wolfe, J., Wiener, L., Lyon, M., & Feudtner, C. (2016). Ethics, emotions, and the skills of talking about progressing disease with terminally ill adolescents: A review. *JAMA Pediatrics, 170*(12), 1216–1223.
- Roter, D. L., Larson, S., Fischer, G. S., Arnold, R. M., & Tulsky, J. A. (2000). Experts practice what they preach: A descriptive study of best and normative practices in end-of-life discussions. *Archives of Internal Medicine, 160*(22), 3477–3485.
- Rushton, C. H., Kaszniak, A. W., & Halifax, J. S. (2013). A framework for understanding moral distress among

palliative care clinicians. *Journal of Palliative Medicine, 16*(9), 1074–1079.

- Sachs, G. A., Shega, J. W., & Cox-Hayley, D. (2004). Barriers to excellent end-of-life care for patients with dementia. *Journal of General Internal Medicine, 19*(10), 1057–1063.
- Sanders, J. J., Curtis, J. R., & Tulsky, J. A. (2018). Achieving goal-concordant care: A conceptual model and approach to measuring serious illness communication and its impact. *Journal of Palliative Medicine, 21*(Suppl. 2), S17–S27.
- Sansbury, B. S., Graves, K., & Scott, W. (2015). Managing traumatic stress responses among clinicians: Individual and organizational tools for self-care. *Trauma, 17*(2), 114–122.
- Saunders, C. (2003). *Watch with me: Inspiration for a life in hospice care*. Mortal Press.
- Schenker, Y., & Arnold, R. M. (2017). Toward palliative care for all patients with advanced cancer. *JAMA Oncology, 3*(11), 1459–1460.
- Schneider, E. C., Sarnak, D. O., Squires, D., Shah, A., & Doty, M. M. (2017). *Mirror, mirror 2017: International comparison reflects flaws and opportunities for better U.S. health care*. The Commonwealth Fund.
- Schulman-Green, D., McCorkle, R., Cherlin, E., Johnson-Hürzeler, R., & Bradley, E. H. (2005). Nurses' communication of prognosis and implications for hospice referral: A study of nurses caring for terminally ill hospitalized patients. *American Journal of Critical Care, 14*(1), 64–70.
- Singer, A. E., Ash, T., Ochotorena, C., Lorenz, K. A., Chong, K., Shreve, S. T., & Ahluwalia, S. C. (2016). A systematic review of family meeting tools in palliative and intensive care settings. *American Journal of Hospice and Palliative Medicine, 33*(8), 797–806.
- Singh, S., Cortez, D., Maynard, D., Cleary, J. F., DuBenske, L., & Campbell, T. C. (2017). Characterizing the nature of scan results discussions: Insights into why patients misunderstand their prognosis. *Journal of Oncology Practice, 13*(3), e231–e239.

- Skulason, B., Hauksdottir, A., Ahcic, K., & Helgason, A. R. (2014). Death talk: Gender differences in talking about one's own impending death. *BMC Palliative Care, 13*, Article 8.
- Stamm, B. H. (2010). *The concise ProQOL manual* (2nd ed.). ProQOL.org.
- Sudore, R. L., & Fried, T. R. (2010). Redefining the "planning" in advance care planning: Preparing for end-of-life decision making. *Annals of Internal Medicine, 153*(4), 256–261.
- Sudore, R. L., Lum, H. D., You, J. J., Hanson, L. C., Meier, D. E., Pantilat, S. Z., Matlock, D. D., Rietjens, J. A. C., Korfage, I. J., Ritchie, C. S., Kutner, J. S., Teno, J. M., Thomas, J., McMahan, R. D., & Heyland, D. K. (2017). Defining advance care planning for adults: A consensus definition from a multidisciplinary Delphi panel. *Journal of Pain and Symptom Management, 53*(5), 821–832.
- Sullivan, A. M., Lakoma, M. D., & Block, S. D. (2003). The status of medical education in end-of-life care: A national report. *Journal of General Internal Medicine, 18*(9), 685–695.
- Sullivan, D. R., Liu, X., Corwin, D. S., Verceles, A. C., McCurdy, M. T., Pate, D. A., Davis, J. M., & Netzer, G. (2012). Learned helplessness among families and surrogate decision makers of patients admitted to medical, surgical, and trauma intensive care units. *Chest, 142*(6), 1440–1446.
- Sveen, J., Eilegard, A., Steineck, G., & Kreicbergs, U. (2014). They still grieve: A nationwide follow-up of young adults 2–9 years after losing a sibling to cancer. *Psycho-Oncology, 23*(6), 658–664.
- Szulanski, G. (1996). Exploring internal stickiness: Impediments to the transfer of best practice within the firm. *Strategic Management Journal, 17*(S2), 27–43.
- Temel, J. S., Greer, J. A., Admane, S., Gallagher, E. R., Jackson, V. A., Lynch, T. J., Lennes, I. T., Dahlin, C. M., & Pirl, W. F. (2011). Longitudinal perceptions of prognosis and goals of therapy in patients with metastatic non-small-cell lung cancer. *Journal of Clinical Oncology, 29*(17), 2319–2326.

- Temel, J. S., Greer, J. A., Muzikansky, A., Gallagher, E. R., Admane, S., Jackson, V. A., Dahlin, C. M., Blinderman, C. D., Jacobsen, J., Pirl, W. F., Billings, J. A., & Lynch, T. J. (2010). Early palliative care for patients with metastatic non-small-cell lung cancer. *New England Journal of Medicine, 363*(8), 733–742.
- Teno, J. M., Gozalo, P. L., Bynum, J. P. W., Leland, N. E., Miller, S. C., Morden, N. E., Scupp, T., Goodman, D. C., & Mor, V. (2013). Change in end-of-life care for Medicare beneficiaries: Site of death, place of care, and health care transitions in 2000, 2005, and 2009. *JAMA, 309*(5), 470–477.
- Tervalon, M., & Murray-García, J. (1998). Cultural humility versus cultural competence: A critical distinction in defining physician training outcomes in multicultural education. *Journal of Health Care for the Poor and Underserved, 9*(2), 117–125.
- Tilden, V. P., Tolle, S. W., Nelson, C. A., & Fields, J. (2001). Family decision making to withdraw life-sustaining treatments from hospitalized patients. *Nursing Research, 50*(2), 105–115.
- Truog, R. D., Campbell, M. L., Curtis, J. R., Haas, C. E., Luce, J. M., Rubenfeld, G. D., Rushton, C. H., & Kaufman, D. C. (2008). Recommendations for end-of-life care in the intensive care unit: A consensus statement by the American College of Critical Care Medicine. *Critical Care Medicine, 36*(3), 953–963.
- Tulsky, J. A. (2005). Beyond advance directives: Importance of communication skills at the end of life. *JAMA, 294*(3), 359–365.
- Tulsky, J. A., Arnold, R. M., Alexander, S. C., Olsen, M. K., Jeffreys, A. S., Rodriguez, K. L., Skinner, C. S., Farrell, D., Abernethy, A. P., & Pollak, K. I. (2011). Enhancing communication between oncologists and patients with a computer-based training program. *Annals of Internal Medicine, 155*(9), 593–601.
- Vachon, M. L. S. (2016). Targeted intervention for family and professional caregivers: Attachment, empathy, and compassion. *Palliative Medicine, 30*(2), 101–103.

- van der Steen, J. T., Radbruch, L., Hertogh, C. M., de Boer, M. E., Hughes, J. C., Larkin, P., Francke, A. L., Jünger, S., Gove, D., Firth, P., Koopmans, R. T., & Volicer, L. (2014). White paper defining optimal palliative care in older people with dementia: A Delphi study and recommendations from the European Association for Palliative Care. *Palliative Medicine, 28*(3), 197–209.
- Vig, E. K., Starks, H., Taylor, J. S., Hopley, E. K., & Fryer-Edwards, K. (2010). Why don't patients enroll in hospice? Can we do anything about it? *Journal of General Internal Medicine, 25*(10), 1009–1019.
- Virdun, C., Luckett, T., Davidson, P. M., & Phillips, J. (2015). Dying in the hospital setting: A systematic review of quantitative studies identifying the elements of end-of-life care that patients and their families rank as being most important. *Palliative Medicine, 29*(9), 774–796.
- Warden, V., Hurley, A. C., & Volicer, L. (2003). Development and psychometric evaluation of the Pain Assessment in Advanced Dementia (PAINAD) scale. *Journal of the American Medical Directors Association, 4*(1), 9–15.
- Washington, K. T., Pike, K. C., Demiris, G., & Parker Oliver, D. (2015). Gaining access to social support on the internet for family caregivers of hospice patients with cancer. *Journal of Hospice and Palliative Nursing, 17*(6), 472–480.
- Way, J., Back, A. L., & Curtis, J. R. (2002). Withdrawing life support and resolution of conflict with families. *BMJ, 325*(7376), 1342–1345.
- Weingarten, K. (2003). *Common shock: Witnessing violence every day—How we are harmed, how we can heal.* New American Library.
- Wheless, M., Lee, J. J., Domenico, H. J., Martin, B. J., Bennett, M. L., Martin, S. F., Berlin, J., Green, J. K., & Agarwal, R. (2023). Factors and barriers to goals-of-care conversations for patients with cancer and inpatient mortality. *JCO Oncology Practice, 19*(9), 767–776.
- Whitebird, R. R., Asche, S. E., Thompson, G. L., Rossom, R., & Heinrich, R. (2013). Stress, burnout, compassion

fatigue, and mental health in hospice workers in Minnesota. *Journal of Palliative Medicine, 16*(12), 1534–1539.

- Widera, E., Anderson, W. G., Santhosh, L., McKee, K. Y., Smith, A. K., & Frank, J. (2020). Family meetings on behalf of patients with serious illness. *New England Journal of Medicine, 383*(11), e71.

- Wiener, L., Zadeh, S., Battles, H., Baird, K., Ballard, E., Osherow, J., & Pao, M. (2012). Allowing adolescents and young adults to plan their end-of-life care. *Pediatrics, 130*(5), 897–905.

- Wittenberg-Lyles, E. M., Goldsmith, J., Sanchez-Reilly, S., & Ragan, S. L. (2008). Communicating a terminal prognosis in a palliative care setting: Deficiencies in current communication training protocols. *Social Science & Medicine, 66*(11), 2356–2365.

- Wittenberg, E., Ferrell, B., Goldsmith, J., Smith, T., Ragan, S. L., Glajchen, M., & Handzo, G. (2015). *Textbook of palliative care communication*. Oxford University Press.

- Wolfe, J., Grier, H. E., Klar, N., Levin, S. B., Ellenbogen, J. M., Salem-Schatz, S., Emanuel, E. J., & Weeks, J. C. (2000). Symptoms and suffering at the end of life in children with cancer. *New England Journal of Medicine, 342*(5), 326–333.

- Wright, A. A., Zhang, B., Ray, A., Mack, J. W., Trice, E., Balboni, T., Mitchell, S. L., Jackson, V. A., Block, S. D., Maciejewski, P. K., & Prigerson, H. G. (2008). Associations between end-of-life discussions, patient mental health, medical care near death, and caregiver bereavement adjustment. *JAMA, 300*(14), 1665–1673.

- Yalom, I. D. (2008). *Staring at the sun: Overcoming the terror of death*. Jossey-Bass.

- Young, E. (2013). Motivational interviewing in end-of-life care. *Psychotherapy.net*.